AF229470

WHAT I NEED FROM YOU

What people with Parkinson's disease want
their care partners and caregivers to
know at every stage of the illness

FELICITY KLOS and **KEVIN KLOS, M.D.**

We dedicate this book to the people with Parkinson's disease and their families who participated in this research project.

We are grateful for their selflessly giving their time and advice to make this book possible.

We especially dedicate this book to Connie and Bill who together demonstrated such love and fortitude as they battled this difficult disease.

CONTENTS

INTRODUCTION

MY FAMILY AND I WERE ATTENDING A PRE-school performance at our local church gymnasium. After a delightful show, my wife and I were exiting the gym behind a couple that were obviously grandparents of one of the preschool students. As a movement disorder specialist, whether in or out of the clinic, you cannot help but examine the way people are walking. I noticed that the grandmother walking in front of me was shuffling her steps and not swinging her arms normally, and also noticed a very subtle tremor in her hands as she walked ahead. They reached a set of four concrete steps leading down to the parking lot. Right in front of me, the woman lost her footing and fell down the steps. Thankfully, she landed on her backside and did not hit her head. The fall happened so fast that neither her husband nor my wife and I could grab her before she fell.

As someone who is used to being a first responder in the hospital, I rushed over to her and provided first aid. I requested she be taken to the local ER to make sure that she had not fractured any bones. I asked her if she would be willing to come to my office for a neurological evaluation. She agreed. I eventually sent her for testing and sat down with her and her husband in my office to review the results.

I said to her, "Mom, you have Parkinson's disease."

This is how she received the official diagnosis. This was the moment when I gained a new role in addition to movement disorder specialist: I was now an official care partner for my mom and her Parkinson's disease (PD). My family, including my daughter Felicity, became care partners for my mom as well. Parkinson's disease affects not only the person with the illness but the entire family.

For a movement disorder specialist, diagnosing a relative with PD is surreal. It is exceedingly difficult to think about all the possible complications and disease progression scenarios you have witnessed with your patients and to then imagine a family member battling the same challenges. Treating PD and finding better treatments became even more of a personal mission.

After my mom was diagnosed with PD, I wanted to become the best care partner I could be for her, so I turned to the literature. However, I had difficulty finding books that provided insights into PD caregiving. Most of the books either provided technical information on the disease itself or were personal memoirs of individual families caring for a loved one with PD. Although these books were interesting and helpful, I needed more information from the people in the trenches taking care of a loved one with PD. I also wanted to know more about what people with PD need in terms of help and support through the disease process, as I knew their needs are different in the early years of PD than they are during the more advanced years.

Then I realized that I had a wealth of knowledge waiting for me in my clinical practice. Why not turn to the people with the disease and the people taking care of them that I see every day? So, that is exactly what I did.

The first project involved interviewing care partners and acquiring all the advice and secrets that they could provide to fellow caregivers. My research and findings were presented in my first book, *You Are a Better Parkinson's Disease Caregiver Than You Think* (2020).

In this book, however, my daughter Felicity and I decided to analyze and write about the second half of the research project, which involved giving hundreds of people with PD in my practice questionnaires about extensive topics. We asked them numerous questions regarding their experience with a care partner or caregiver and asked them for advice that we could share with others. The questionnaires were completed by the patient alone in the clinic and were anonymous; this was to avoid a care partner or caregiver influencing their answers. We assured them that we would not discuss their answers with them or their family members so that the information would remain private. However, they did consent to us using this information in this current book.

Next, we held advisory board meetings where Felicity and I interviewed a small group of patients, again without their caregiver or family member present so that they could speak candidly and in private. Each advisory board consisted of people at the same stage of PD. We also divided the groups by gender so that we could identify any particular issues that were unique to either gender.

We learned directly from people with Parkinson's disease about their opinions on all aspects of caregiving. (We did not include individuals suffering from dementia since they would not be able to provide us with accurate or reliable information.) We wanted to learn what the patient actually needs from their care partner and/or caregiver at each stage of the illness. We wanted to learn from the patients themselves how they prefer to be treated during the variety of challenges they face throughout the disease process. They shared with us what they thought were helpful and successful approaches to their problems and what not to do in certain situations. We evaluated their responses based on their stage of the disease. We specifically analyzed different responses by age, gender, and personality type.

Jared's Story

"I'm so confused about how best to help my wife with her Parkinson's disease," says Jared. Jared and his wife have been married for over fifty years. "When I worked as an engineer, everything that I did was organized and systematic, and the outcomes were predictable. Now, in my new job as a caregiver, I feel lost! I don't know what to do to help her. I can't read her mind! She is annoyed with my help at times, yet open to my caring at other times. I get so much conflicting advice from the members of our support group. Even when I search the internet for suggestions, I end up increasingly confused."

Perhaps you, like Jared, are living with the challenge of being a care partner or caregiver for a loved one with PD. You may feel like you have too much on your plate. You desperately want to love and care for your loved one as much as is humanly possible, but maybe at times you feel insecure about the best approach to take in helping your loved one. You may at times want your loved one to remain as independent as possible, so you let them manage certain tasks without saying a word or without intervening. Then there are times when you feel you just need to jump in and help. However, your loved one's response may not always be the same and may not be what you anticipated. You have found yourself facing a major challenge: you have taken on a job that you did not apply for and you have no formal training. But this is now a full-time 24/7 job—and it is becoming progressively more difficult.

Caregiving is one of the most difficult jobs on the planet. It is a full-time job that, like parenting, can involve all hours of the day and night. There is stress due to constantly worrying about your loved one and your family. You may become exhausted and overwhelmed. Your sleep habits may change, resulting in even more fatigue, increased irritation, and sometimes anger. You may not be able to participate in the activities or hobbies you enjoy. Relationships may change as you are not able to spend time away from your caring responsibilities. Friendships may dwindle due to a lack of attention and time spent together. Even the relationship with your loved one with PD may change. It is common for a married couple to find their relationship has changed from *loving partners to a parent-child dynamic.* It is especially hard to watch the disease progressively change your loved one's health, as PD causes the degeneration of mental and physical functions. You find yourself having to learn new medical terms, provide new medications, and see your loved one undergo new procedures to manage PD.

> *Caregiving is one of the most*
> *difficult jobs on the planet.*

More of us are now in the position of having to care for a loved one with Parkinson's disease, as the incidence of PD is rising exponentially worldwide. The World Health Organization has estimated that the prevalence of Parkinson's disease has doubled over the last twenty-five years. The number of people diagnosed with PD worldwide is expected to continue to rise exponentially, with over ten million people affected. Spouses, adult children, and other family members suddenly find themselves caregiving for an illness that they have heard of but know truly little about. These individuals certainly have no experience in caregiving and lack insights into how to effectively do so.

When we find ourselves in the caregiving role, we often wonder, "Am I doing this right?" Countless care partners and caregivers over the years have asked me, "What is the right way to …." You can search the internet and bookstores to find caregiving books for people with Parkinson's disease and certainly you will find books that describe a family's experience with the disease or technical information about the disease itself. However, you will not find a manual with step-by-step instructions or with advice on how to actually address the myriad issues that arise along the course of the disease. I know this because when I became a care partner, I could not find the resources I was looking for to help my mom manage her Parkinson's disease.

> *You can search the internet and bookstores*
> *to find caregiving books for people with*
> *Parkinson's disease, but you will not find a*
> *manual with step-by-step instructions.*

A Common Approach to PD Caregiving

Here is a common scenario involving family members of a newly diagnosed person with PD. After your loved one has received the diagnosis and has shared it with you and those family members and friends they wish to tell, you find yourself dealing with several issues. You are often wondering, "How much does my loved one wish to talk about

PD on a daily basis? Is it better for me to pretend that they don't have the diagnosis and go on with life 'as usual'? Should I do some research on the illness and look at new treatments and present my findings to my loved one on an ongoing basis? Will this constant reminder of the illness cause my loved one to get depressed and discouraged? Does my loved one wish I would just ignore PD altogether and look the other way? How much should I be encouraging them to follow the advice of their healthcare provider when it comes to lifestyle issues, including exercise, diet, and sleep?" In the end, you might think, "I certainly don't want to be a nag."

It is also common for people in the early stages of PD to downplay their symptoms or to seem uninterested in discussing the symptoms, emotions, and fears that they are experiencing because they do not want to alarm or worry you, even though it would greatly help for them to discuss them with someone. You might ask yourself, "Do I ask them if they have taken their medication today and, if they did, did they take it on time? Do I need to remind them or just leave them alone and trust that they are managing their medication independently? Does it bother them if I ask if they took their medicine today?"

Years later, as they approach the more advanced stages of the disease, new challenges arise. By now they have collaborated with a physical therapist and/or speech therapist who provide them with detailed recommendations on performing day-to-day movements as well as stretching and exercise. These therapists may have encouraged you to remind your loved one to stand up straight, take big steps when they walk, pull their shoulders back for better posture, speak with intent, and keep their head up when talking to others, among other helpful advice. "Should I continuously remind my loved one to do these things throughout the day? Does this help them? Why do they keep forgetting these techniques and why is it so difficult to get them to exercise?" Of course, they do know how important these exercises are to fighting the disease and they have been told by so many healthcare specialists to do them every day.

Typically, such challenges strain your relationship with your loved one with PD, especially as it begins to shift to a parent-child type of relationship and you begin treating your loved one like a child. You find yourself repeating, "Do this… do that… and don't forget to do this…."

In many cases, your loved one with PD may become more withdrawn and less vocal. As communication breaks down, a caregiver who has assumed more of the day-to-day demands may receive no feedback at all from their loved one. Now you are really beginning to wonder if you are being helpful at all. Yet you persist because you feel it is the right thing to do. You must just get the job done and, as a parent, you are going to do it your way and hope that it is the best way.

Conducting Research for This Book

The people with PD who participated in this project were a diverse group. There were slightly more men than women and ranged in age from forty-two to their late eighties. None of the people with PD showed evidence of dementia. They all had the cognitive ability to share their opinions and thoughts about their experience with PD and with their care partner or caregiver. None were living in an institution, so we could discuss issues that were related to caregiving at home with families. (Most people reading this book are actively helping a loved one with PD and are not necessarily part of the staff working in a nursing facility.) The majority of those with advanced PD were retired or disabled, while many in the early-stage of PD were still working full- or part-time jobs. The participants were also from diverse racial and ethnic backgrounds and espoused a variety of religions, although some had quit practicing their faith tradition.

In this project, we aimed to evaluate whether personality type may play a role in the information and advice that we received. Although psychiatrists have described and elucidated many personality types, we decided to keep it simple and focus on two personality types: Type A and Type B. We explained to the participants that a Type A person is often highly organized, extremely ambitious, sometimes impatient, and always prefers to be in charge or in control. Meanwhile, a *Type B personality is* more passive and relaxed, and may be less organized and less competitive. They tend to worry less about who wins the competition but instead just enjoy playing the game. They also tend to be more patient and flexible. The participants were asked to identify with one of these personality types for the purpose of our research.

When we think about caregiving as a job, we might ask ourselves several questions. "How do we know if we are doing a decent job? Who should judge how we are doing as caregivers?"

Of course it is not necessary to be graded on job performance: we are not receiving a paycheck or bonus for our work. Ultimately, you are free to care for another human being as you wish. However, most of my patients with PD have caregivers who thoughtfully would like to know if they are doing a respectable job, and thus they seek approval from their healthcare provider, family, friends, and fellow caregivers whom they encounter at support groups or meetings. Realistically, the only person's opinion that we should be interested in for purposes of evaluating our performance is our loved one with Parkinson's disease.

They are the target of our service and their evaluation of us is the most important evaluation we should receive.

This book provides you with the opinions of a large group of people with PD to help guide your decisions as you manage different challenges and issues along your challenging caregiving journey.

> *The only person's opinion that we should be interested in for evaluating our performance is our loved one with Parkinson's disease.*

In this book, we offer the answers and advice from our advisory boards provided by the people with PD. We hope this information helps you approach your role as a care partner or caregiver with more confidence and peace. This book is full of the wisdom that people with PD shared with us. You will find valuable insights into the world of caregiving directly from the people who need your love and support. They taught us many lessons about how to help them along their difficult journey, and we hope that these lessons will also be helpful to you as you continue assisting your loved one with PD.

Chapter 1

WORRY ABOUT A PARKINSON FUTURE

YOU WOULD NOT BE HUMAN IF YOU DID NOT have a lot of worries or anxiety about living with a diagnosis of Parkinson's disease. However, these worries may change as the disease progresses, and new fears may be added along the way. So, we wanted to better understand the worries that people with PD experience at different stages of the illness. And we were curious if the worries differ between men and women or between different personality types. Undoubtedly, people at different ages and stages of life will have specific worries depending on their personal circumstances.

We also wanted to know how the person with PD felt about their care partner or caregiver responding to these fears. What approach did they prefer? What techniques should be avoided? Ultimately, our hope was to gain insights into how best to support our loved ones along their journey and perhaps also lessen their burden of anxiety.

Talking About PD

We began with individuals in the early stages of PD. We wanted to know their opinions on whether the care partner should talk about the disease with them. Do they mind if the care partner discusses the disease's progression or complications with them? Perhaps the person with PD prefers not to discuss this in order to reduce their anxiety. Obviously, the care partner will have their own anxiety about how PD will affect their loved one and how it will affect them. But, should the care partner keep these anxieties hidden from their loved one with PD?

We asked our people with PD about this issue of talking about the disease in its early stages. Overall, 65% of the people with PD preferred that the care partner openly talk about the disease and how it progresses. Of this 65%, there was no difference in gender or personality type. As for the 35% who did not want to discuss the disease or its progression, more of these individuals were women and identified as Type A personalities. The age of the person with PD did not affect their opinion on this topic.

Clearly, the group was closely split on their opinion of this question. Perhaps some type A personalities may prefer to avoid a discussion because they feel less in control. However, it is best to talk to your loved one with PD regarding their personal opinion on this topic. Some individuals may gain reassurance in knowing more about the disease and having fewer questions swirling in their mind. They may also appreciate the research you conduct on your own and which you share with them. This may demonstrate to them that you care about arming yourself with valuable information and understanding so that together you may be better equipped to manage the challenges ahead.

Next, we wanted to know what fears or anxieties were foremost in the minds of people in the early stages of PD. They reported four major fears or worries about their future with PD. By far, the number one worry reported by over two-thirds of the group was the loss of independence. Indeed, PD leads to progressive physical disabilities that require more outside help in performing daily functions. For instance, a person with PD may need help getting out of a chair, in and out of bed, walking, and taking care of their personal needs. PD may also lead to cognitive impairment, which makes it difficult for individuals to oversee their own affairs, drive a vehicle, and pursue work or hobbies.

The second worry was related to disease complications. These complications included a multitude of symptoms, cognitive impairment or dementia, concerns about how the disease may affect other organs besides the brain, concerns about mobility, and the adverse effects of the medications and treatments required. Many of these concerns stemmed from what an individual had heard about the condition or information they had read on the internet or in a book.

The third most common fear was being a burden to others. People with PD feared the idea that their loved one would become physically and mentally exhausted. They even feared their loved one would become injured for example when trying to lift them from the floor after a fall. They feared they were holding their family back from their activities, social interactions and plans, and would eventually desire participating in them.

Lastly, the fourth most common worry was that eventually the medications would stop working and that no effective treatment would be left to help them. Unfortunately, there are many myths and misconceptions on the internet and in books, and sometimes even healthcare specialists help perpetuate these fears.

Top Four Fears of Early-Stage People with PD:

1. Loss of independence

2. Disease complications

3. A burden to others

4. Treatments may stop working

Autumn's Story

Autumn was within the first year of being diagnosed with PD. As she began reading books about PD, she developed many concerns about the disease and what might develop over the upcoming years. She listened to podcasts and webinars about the complications of PD and the unmet challenges of the disease progression. All of this information exacerbated her fears.

Autumn's husband, meanwhile, took a different approach. He thought that what they should know about PD would be explained to them by their doctor and thus he did not feel compelled to conduct additional research on his own. The couple went on with their life with PD and although Autumn's anxiety remained hidden, it was greatly affecting her quality of life.

Autumn shared with me that she joined a local support group, hoping the group would provide her with enough information and resources to calm her fears. She explained that the facilitator asked each person at the meeting to share their feelings, questions, and concerns with the group. Each person shared different problems and concerns, many of which Autumn had never heard about or experienced herself. And although she waited for the group to produce some solution or recommendation regarding how to deal with these issues, none were provided. Instead, she walked away with elevated anxiety and increased fears about the future. And when she expressed her concerns, one woman told her, "Honey, it's only going to get worse!" What a blow this was to hear.

Autumn eventually stopped going to this support group. She shared with me that the best solution for her in finding a way to deal with her anxiety and fears about the disease was to visit with her movement disorder specialist. When she was given valuable information about her specific condition and how the illness was progressing for her, her anxieties lessened. The reassurances her specialist provided comforted her considerably, knowing that someone would be there to help her through any grim times. Autumn also received a few immensely helpful books from a national PD organization and these provided helpful tips for dealing with the issues and concerns troubling her mind.

Worry About the Health of the Care Partner

We then asked patients in the early stages of PD if they were worried about their care partner's health being compromised by their role as a caregiver for them. 60% of the people with PD were not particularly worried about the health of their care partner being compromised by caring for them, while 40% were quite worried about whether their care partner would be healthy and strong enough to care for them in the later stages of the disease. Older respondents had a higher likelihood of having medical conditions that raised this concern, while gender and personality type did not play a role in how this question was answered.

Although it is wonderful that 40% of people with PD do not report any anxiety or fear about their caregiver's health being compromised due to their caregiving role, the care partner should not assume that their loved one is in this camp! It is important to talk to your loved one about any concerns they might have about your medical condition and physical and mental strength to assist them. Help them communicate their fears to you and you will both benefit.

Do not just placate them by saying, "I'll be fine" or "I'll always be here for you." Instead, show them you are concerned about your own health and strength to be there for them. Make sure you stay up to date on seeing your healthcare providers regularly. Get regular check-ups and testing done as necessary. Try to follow a healthy diet, get plenty of sleep, and pursue an exercise routine. Share this plan with your loved one so they feel more confident that you are doing your part to stay strong and healthy during this journey you are taking together. They want you to be well-equipped to be there for them in the future.

In the more advanced stages, as patients increasingly lose independence, the shift of anxiety moves toward disease complications and worry about potential treatment failures. The second major concern was being a burden to others. At least half of those with advanced PD were worried about being a burden to others. This did not vary by personality type or gender. Most were worried about the health of their caregiver and whether that caregiver would be able to continue caring for them over the long term.

Don's Story

Don was in the sixth year of PD when he noticed a subtle change in his cognitive performance. Don shared how he would have difficulty producing the right word while speaking and having to stop and awkwardly pause while trying to find it. He would tell people, "I'm having a Parkinson moment, please excuse me."

Don's cognitive problems continued to worsen over the year with not just word finding and forgetting a name: there were now higher-level challenges involving decisions and calculations. He described standing at the check-out counter at the grocery store (he was shopping alone that day) and the clerk giving him the total amount owed for his purchases. As Don dug into his wallet for cash, he realized that his brain was freezing up and he could not count the bills to produce the correct amount owing. He looked at the long line of people behind him impatiently waiting for him to move along. The stress of everyone waiting on him to pay the bill only made matters worse for his cognitive challenge. He finally handed his wallet to the clerk and asked the clerk to take out the correct amount to pay his bill. He was deeply embarrassed by his cognitive lapse.

When Don returned home, he did some searching on the internet about these cognitive challenges: by the end of his research, he was now convinced that he had dementia. He thought, "I'm in the end stages of PD if I have dementia already!" His anxiety level was through the roof and he lost all confidence in himself and hope for the future.

Don came into the clinic and told me about what had happened to him. We decided to try a medication that was designed for treating cognitive impairment in PD. He did not even know that a treatment existed for this condition and was happy to learn about it. Don took the starting dose of the medication for a month, and when he returned to clinic a month later, he told me the great news that his cognitive problems had greatly improved. He told me that he was much better in his conversations with people and only rarely had problems producing the word or idea he wished to express. He returned to shopping alone at the grocery store and had no trouble at all paying the bill.

Don told me that the key to helping his fears about developing dementia and being in the late stage of the disease was talking to me about the problem and receiving a treatment. He now realized that he was not at the end and could function better. He understood that PD is treatable and that seeing his healthcare provider gave him the potential to feel better.

Support for Our Loved One

There are many ways that we can help support our loved one with Parkinson's disease and alleviate these fears. If the person with PD sees that we are taking care of our own health by means of a healthy diet, exercise, and getting plenty of sleep and support, this will reduce their anxiety. We should have regular check-ups with our healthcare providers and share the results with them, where appropriate, to ease their concerns. We want them to maintain confidence that the care partner and caregiver will be there to support them over the long haul and that a backup plan is in place should something happen to them, or if they need more help. Each party should communicate their fears and anxieties to each other. If a specific plan to reduce these anxieties becomes obvious, then certainly follow this plan. Sometimes just having a plan in place, even if the solution is not known yet, may calm some of these anxieties.

Putting on Your Oxygen Mask First

As a care partner or caregiver, it is essential that you manage any anxiety symptoms that you may be experiencing first before looking to help your loved one with PD. It is exceedingly difficult to calm the fears and anxieties of your loved one if you are full of fear and anxiety yourself. Even if you think you can hide your anxiety or keep your fears secret from your loved one, they know how to read your looks and your behaviors, and listen to your tone of voice. It is quite easy for a loved one to pick up on these non-verbal cues that express worry and concern, which in turn may elevate their anxiety levels.

There is no doubt an extensive list of worries and/or fears that a care partner or caregiver could produce when caring for a loved one with PD. These worries can include present situation worries such as dealing with day-to-day challenges. Worries may also include concerns about the future both for your loved one as well as yourself. It does not take long for someone dwelling on all of the potential future scenarios for anxiety levels to go through the roof.

> *Sometimes, just having a plan in place,*
> *even if the solution is not known yet,*
> *may calm some of these anxieties.*

Advice on Reducing Anxiety

One of the best ways to get a handle on your anxiety and fears is to start a journal. In this journal, write down a specific fear or concern at the top of a page. Beneath the topic heading, write down each feared scenario related to that concern. Think of all the possible negative results that could happen and write them down. Next, think of all of the opposite positive outcomes that could result in the future related to that topic. Writing all this down helps free your mind, creating a catharsis. Now, tell yourself that you are going to leave these concerns in the book and empty your mind of such wasteful thoughts. Start a new page for each fear or concern that presents itself along the way, even if you have written about it before. Envision yourself vacuuming out the garbage from your mind and emptying it onto the paper. We must vacuum our homes repeatedly as new trash accumulates, and we need to repeat the vacuuming out of our fears and concerns as well. It is better to remove fears instead of just suppressing them in your mind.

Equally effective is meeting with a counselor or friend willing to listen and sharing your concerns with them.

At the end of each page filled with scenarios, try to write one to three things for which you are grateful. It does not necessarily have to be "grateful for your loved one with PD." It can be gratitude for beautiful weather today or thankful that someone in your life loves you unconditionally. Just write down some things that you are grateful for and do not worry about repeating some of the same ideas.

Your next step is to occupy your mind with a different topic than the fear or worry you were just ruminating over. Stay focused on the other duties you have for the day and week to come. Plan out what you need to do to better support your loved one with PD. Occupying your mind with more objective thoughts and tasks will refocus you away from the anxiety. Move forward with the plan and try to incorporate time with other people. This may be with your loved one with PD or other people in your life. Being around other people that we care about will often help us feel better about our anxieties and bring some joy back into our lives. To avoid relapsing into your recent fears, you may have to be careful about spending too much time with negative people or people who are filled with fear and anxiety.

Another technique is to practice what is called the physiologic "sigh." This breathing technique allows a person to rapidly calm down their nervous system and relax both mind and body. This breathing pattern consists of taking in a deep breath, then trying to inhale a second deep breath immediately at the end of the first deep breath to maximize all the air that can get into your lungs. Next, slowly exhale the air over the next three to four seconds and feel the tension releasing from your body. Repeat this process two more times only and you should feel calmer and less anxious.

Lastly, another wonderful way to curb anxiety and fear is through your spirituality. People who are religious will turn to their faith in God. They will turn to prayer to calm both mind and body and refocus their thoughts on a higher being and away from themselves. Many believers find great comfort and support in their religious community. The belief that there is a place that we will go to one day, one that is free of suffering and pain yet full of love and happiness for eternity, provides great comfort during even the most trying times. If you have fallen away from your faith, perhaps rethinking your spiritual life may be a step in the direction of calming your fears and stress levels, as well as possibly helping your loved one with PD move in the same direction, thereby calming their fears and anxieties as well.

Tips for minimizing common anxieties:

- Start a journal

- Refocus on current tasks or other topics

- Minimize time with negative people
  that elevate anxiety levels

- Use breathing techniques to
  calm the nervous system

- Seek calm through spiritual practice

Caregiver Fears and Anxieties Compared to Their Loved One with PD

We learned in the first part of the project, as we surveyed caregivers, that their anxiety could be divided into two categories: the first was concern for the patient and the second was concern about their own future. This was not much different from the anxieties reported by those with PD, who also had fears about themselves in relation to the progression of the disease as well as fears about how they would affect others in being a burden to them in the future.

In our previous book, *You Are a Better PD Caregiver Than You Think*, caregivers were concerned that they may not be supportive enough for their loved ones now or in the future. They fear that they are not listening enough to the patient's concerns. Interestingly, none of the people with PD had this concern at all. None expressed a concern that their care partner or caregiver would not be supportive enough or love them enough through the battle. This did not even seem to cross their mind as a possibility. So, care partners and caregivers should avoid putting excessive pressure on themselves. Instead, realize you will always support your loved one to the best of your ability. This level of support will always be optimal for their loved one because the love is coming from you, not someone else.

Care partners and caregivers do not have to solve all the problems that people with PD experience. Focus on finding resources and information that may help them. Sometimes, people with PD just need someone to listen to them. They want to be heard, and especially by a loving and empathetic care partner. It is often therapeutic for people with PD to verbalize their feelings, concerns, and anxieties. It helps them to feel validated and to know that their symptoms are real.

> *Your level of support will always be optimal for your loved one because the love is coming from you, not someone else.*

Chapter 2

NAGGING IS TOUGH ON A RELATIONSHIP

Mark's Story

Mark attended one of our advisory meetings. He shared a story with us that illustrates a common scenario that often creates significant strife in relationships. Mark was diagnosed with PD about twelve years ago, while he was still working. The progression of his PD resulted in enough disability that Mark could no longer fulfill his work duties. Mark had never pursued any hobbies outside of work. He was not an athlete and never enjoyed exercise.

Mark's wife watched him transition from being busy at work each day to becoming a lazy person. The only exercise that Mark admitted to doing was occasionally walking the dog around the block, although this was not often or consistent.

Mark's wife had spent extensive time over the years researching PD on the internet, reading books, and attending educational seminars. She understood how important diet and exercise are to managing

PD. For some years, she tried not to nag him about exercising and watching his diet. She tried subtle and not-so-subtle techniques to encourage him to exercise. She would ask the neurologist, at Mark's appointments, to convince him to start exercising. She grew increasingly concerned about him as she watched him get weaker and weaker. She noted his balance was much worse: he suffered several falls resulting in minor injuries. She was finally so frustrated that she could no longer hold back: she now feared for his health.

Mark shared with us the strain being placed on his marriage. We asked him about what he wished his care partner would change or do differently. Mark immediately said, "I want her to stop nagging me all day long!"

Mark felt that his wife was constantly nagging him to exercise and to start a hobby. She would plead with him to find something that he might be interested in doing so he would get off the couch. Mark found lots of ways to dismiss her, or sometimes he would offer empty promises that he would start a program but then never follow through. Mark grew increasingly resentful of his wife. He just could not stand her nagging. He admitted that on many days, the nagging encouraged him to passive-aggressively refrain from exercising just to spite her. He became increasingly irritable and at times angry. He had lost any motivation to become involved with anything productive. He did not want to do any chores at home. His marriage was strained and all the joy in his relationship with his wife was lost. Eventually, they stopped communicating with each other and became distant roommates instead of a happily married couple.

Nagging

Nagging is a common problem in many families dealing with PD, and
PD creates the perfect opportunity for nagging to arise. Here we have
a condition that robs an individual of their motivation and desire for
most activities, but especially activities such as exercise. It is difficult
for people with PD to motivate themselves for activities like exercise
that may result in physical exertion, discomfort, and at times suffering. Meanwhile, a loved one and other family members are wishing
so strongly for the optimum health of their loved one with PD. They
are worried about the progression and disability that will likely result.
They want to help their loved one in any way they can, but they are
stuck because they cannot exercise for them. They cannot pursue hobbies, activities, and social interactions for them. They cannot always
force them to eat a certain way or take big steps all the time. They feel
guilty and at times ashamed of the way they nag their loved one, but
they do not always know how to approach this issue in a positive and
beneficial way.

The dictionary states that nagging is "constantly harassing someone to do something" (Oxford Language Dictionary online). When
we read this definition, we are struck by the word "harassing." I know
that when I nag my loved one, I do not mean to harass them. This
violent-sounding word suggests a verbal assault, one which I never
intended. To me, nagging consists of simple reminders, which, in my

mind, are offered to elicit a positive outcome. This reminder is backed by a genuine interest in the well-being of my loved one; otherwise, I would not put the effort into repeating the request.

To the person with PD, however, the word harass may sound like an excellent choice. This may truly be how they feel about the verbal reminders and suggestions offered repeatedly. Through the struggles of the day, reminders about anything could simply build up frustration, shame, and feelings of anger toward their loved one. Some of my patients admit to passive-aggressive responses to the nagging by purposely not performing the desired task, just boomerang the frustration back to their partner. Other people with PD just simply forget repeatedly to perform the desired task. Reasons for this may include short-term memory loss, changes in judgment related to the frontal lobe executive dysfunction of the disease, medication's adverse effects, poor sleep quality, and others. Many of the problems that we nag about, such as posture, short steps, and a soft voice, are automatic functions of the brain that people with PD do not actively think about.

As a care partner or caregiver, we are not sure if the nagging that we do is helpful to our loved one with PD or is counterproductive. This is especially true when there is no communication or feedback from our loved one to help us understand their feelings about the issue. We often do not take the time to ask how they feel about our repeated requests, and even if we do ask, we cannot be sure that their response is sincerely honest.

Some of the more common ways that we nag our loved one with Parkinson's disease include reminders about their physical performance. This often stems from the advice given to our loved one by the physical therapist, for example. We hear the physical therapist reminding our loved one to stand up straight when they walk. We hear them emphasizing "big steps" and "make your arm swing." We hear the speech therapist remind our loved one to "speak louder" or "speak with intent." As the care partner, we now feel that we have the license to reiterate these reminders at home. We see ourselves as home extensions of these therapists and therefore we think we need to continue spreading the message.

We also hear about the importance of exercise for our loved ones. The healthcare providers and movement disorder specialists, along with the therapists, emphasize the need for exercise and all its benefits. In fact, in our clinic, we even go so far as equating exercise to a form of medication. We tell our patients that exercise is a "have to" as part of PD treatment and must form a routine part of their schedule.

One of the cruel aspects of having PD is that dopamine levels are lower in the brain, resulting in a lack of motivation. Then we tell the patient they must have the motivation each day to exercise—when this is the last thing they want to do. For many people with PD, exercise is uncomfortable. The muscle pain and stiffness make exercising difficult. Exercise for anyone can bring about some level of discomfort because of our weakness and deconditioning. Patients get winded easily and tired at the start of their exercise routine. Who would want to continue this torture day in and day out?

When we talk to care partners and caregivers, they are often unsure if they should "nag" about these issues daily. Some do not even worry about whether their partner wishes to be nagged or not: they just do so regardless. This nagging, at its root, aims to create for the caregiver some kind of order to what seems like an unmanaged situation.

In our research, we decided to ask our patients with PD how they felt about their caregiver nagging them about specific issues. We analyzed the responses according to PD stage, responses by men versus women, responses based on personality type, and response by age.

Nagging About Exercise

For the patients with early PD, we were not surprised to find an equal split regarding whether the patients wanted to be reminded (or encouraged) to exercise. The men in our group were much more likely to express the desire for their care partner to encourage them to exercise, while the women were less thrilled about the reminders. A Type B personality individual was less likely to want reminders, as were the younger patients. The older the patient, the more likely they were to prefer gentle reminders to exercise.

Most patients with advanced PD wished to be nagged about exercising. In this group, both men and women were equally thrilled about the reminders. Personality type did not play a role in their interest in nagging about exercise.

Interestingly, the longer one had PD and the older the individual was, the more they appreciated the reminders about exercising. This suggests that exercise was ultimately beneficial to the patient, and because these patients are more prone to suffer from apathy as they age and experience PD, these reminders were helpful.

Regardless of the stage of the disease, there appears to be an evenly divided split on how people with PD feel about nagging about exercise. It is important that the care partner and caregiver communicate about this issue. Find out if your loved one wants you to be their cheerleader and to encourage them to keep up their exercise program consistently. Find out how they want you to remind them. Perhaps instead of saying, "Did you exercise today?" you might consider asking, "What is your plan today for exercise?" Or you could ask, "What time are you exercising today? I'd like to exercise too!" Perhaps you can find a way to exercise together.

We think it is also important to keep in mind that PD will commonly cause people to have good and bad days with their symptoms. We all have a bad day now and again. However, with PD, bad days may prevail. On these bad days, a person with PD will struggle to perform physically and may not be able to exercise at their usual intensity and performance level. Furthermore, on bad days the mental symptoms, especially apathy, may be intensified, making motivation to exercise difficult. A care partner and caregiver should be aware of these situations and be patient with their loved one. Realize that missing a day here and there will not matter to the long-term outcome. However, if your loved one is not exercising for a longer stretch of time, then it may be best to reach out to the healthcare provider to determine if medications may need to be adjusted so that exercise may resume.

Nagging About Taking "Big Steps"

We then asked our group of people with PD how they specifically felt about their partner asking them to take bigger steps when they walk. We know that taking bigger steps repetitively helps to curtail the automatic tendency to take short steps, and short steps create problems with our balance and may lead to falls. To maintain better walking and balance, a longer stride is necessary.

Most of our early-stage PD patients, 85%, stated that they were not bothered when their care partner reminded them to take big steps. There was no difference in gender or personality type for the 15% that were bothered by the nagging. The individual bothered by the nagging tended to be those who were closer to the time of their PD diagnosis, especially those within the first five years of the illness. Perhaps this group did not realize how much of a problem they had with their steps and did not want to be reminded of such limitations.

In the advanced PD group, 91% reported that it was no bother to them to be reminded to take big steps. Of the 9% bothered by this type of nagging, women were three times more likely to be bothered, as were the Type A personalities. Age and years with PD did not seem to have influence in this group.

Nagging About "Standing Up Straight"

As PD progresses, bad posture becomes increasingly an issue. The progressive weakness of the back muscles contribute to the posture flexing forward. A stooped posture creates a mechanical disadvantage when taking normal-sized steps. The more we stoop, the more we shuffle our feet while walking.

In the early PD group, 78% had no objection to this specific nagging about standing up straight. Of the 22% who were bothered by the nagging, men were more likely than women to be bothered. The people identifying as Type B personalities and having a longer-duration PD were less likely to be bothered by the nagging.

In the advanced PD group, 88% of the patients reported having no objection to the nagging about posture. However, of the 12% that were bothered by the nagging, all of them happened to be men. There was no significant difference in personality type or age for this group.

Nagging About "Speak Up and With Intent"

Universally, people with PD experience a progressive change in their voice, which becomes softer and softer over time. In many, articulation will break down, causing the listener to have more difficulty understanding the words. Now caregivers find themselves repeating, "What did you say?"

Parkinson's disease changes the automatic process of taking in a deep breath and forcing the air out of the lungs to produce a strong, loud voice. As the breaths become shallower as the disease progresses, speech volume continues to diminish. We see patients that have reached a stage at which they speak in a mere whisper due to loss of power in the vocal production.

Compounding the problem of low volume is a change in auditory perception that commonly results from PD. People with PD will hear their voice and think they are speaking loud enough for everyone to hear them. Unfortunately, the true volume of their speech *is* below normal decibel readings for conversational speech. This creates the need for people to gently inform their loved one that they are speaking in too low a volume.

We asked our people with PD how they felt about being nagged to speak out louder. In the early PD group, 75% were not bothered by the nagging. For those who did not want to be told to speak up louder and with intent, there was no difference in gender, personality type, or age. In the advanced PD group, 88% were not bothered by this type of nagging. There was no difference in gender, personality, years with PD, or age in the 12% that were bothered.

The majority did not have a problem with these reminders, especially as the disease advanced. When a person with PD repeated something using a louder voice, they were often able to speak much louder and much clearer.

Some of the caregivers will remark that their loved one with PD communicates better at the doctor's office than at home. Naturally, people with PD are more relaxed and comfortable at home with their family. They do not have to concentrate or put as much effort into communicating and thus they let the automatic process of speaking softly and slowly prevail. The automatic process of speaking with PD is a progressively softer voice with poor articulation. Compounding the communication challenge may be the reduced hearing of their aging caregiver.

People With PD's Advice on Nagging

We asked our patients for some solutions to suggest to the care partner or caregiver regarding minimizing nagging but still encouraging patients to pursue exercise. First, they wanted their loved ones to discuss expectations with them. The person with PD wanted to be able to communicate how much exercise and what type of exercise they felt comfortable pursuing at any point in the illness. They wanted to know what the expectations of the care partner or caregiver were so they could discuss whether this was a realistic goal at this point.

Second, the patient did not want to be criticized for their current exercise pattern. They did not feel good about feeling ashamed of any lack of consistency with their exercising. They felt like their loved one should lead by example. If their loved one is going to nag about exercise yet never do any exercise themselves, the suggestion falls somewhat flat and becomes irritating. The patient did not want the caregiver to automatically jump to the conclusion that they were being lazy or pathetic when they did not exercise. There may be times when their medication is not working as well, or when the disease is flaring up and they are more uncomfortable or suffer more pain. The muscles may be weak on certain days, which limits their success in the exercise session.

Third, it is often beneficial to have an exercise partner to keep up the motivation and prevent nagging. If you, as the care partner or caregiver, exercise with them (instead of nagging), you can simply schedule an exercise session together and accomplish the task.

Fourth, the person with PD often felt better about the nagging when they received from their loved one some sort of appreciation for their accomplishment. This could be a simple verbal affirmation or a bigger reward, perhaps after completing so many days or months of exercise. Tell them how proud of them you are when they string together a few exercises each day for weeks or months at a time.

Fourth, be kind to your loved one when you remind them about exercise. Remind them in a positive and encouraging way. Pay attention to the "right time" to remind them, not when they are struggling with something else or feel down about their symptoms or situation. Remember that it is not your job to control them but rather to be an encouraging partner. What they ultimately decide to do is their choice and we must accept this. Even if we think we would do things differently if we had PD, we cannot expect our loved one to do everything exactly as we think we would in their situation. The more we nag, the more we may eventually feel burned out. Fewer frequent reminders will help prevent adding to caregiver burnout, whereas more frequent nagging will often lead to a higher chance of arguments with your loved one.

Advice on limiting nagging:

- Discuss the expectations of both parties

- Do not criticize

- Find an exercise partner

- Remind with kindness

- Affirm positive responses and celebrate accomplishments

Nagging and Relationships

Nagging may become a major strain on a relationship. The person targeted by the nagging may feel unappreciated. As a care partner or caregiver, we need to learn strategies to minimize nagging and instead find ways to encourage exercise and physical behaviors that can help our loved one. In most cases, the nagging does not end up changing the behavior. Although your loved one may respond to you at that moment, this does not guarantee they will do so indefinitely.

People with PD consistently reported that if the care partner or caregiver used a positive and empathetic tone, perhaps by first saying "Please" before the request is made, then the person receiving the request would be less bothered. A gentle reminder is preferred—and without repetition. Such daily repetition is not helpful and may generate frustration and anger in the person with PD. Give the patient a chance to respond to the request and honor their decision regarding how they wish to respond.

William's Story

William shared with us some of the solutions that he and his wife agreed upon in dealing with nagging. For years, William had grown very irritated with his wife every time she reminded him to exercise or to stand up straight and take bigger steps. She herself had also grown frustrated and irritated that she had to keep reminding William about these issues. She would tell me, "Why doesn't he just remember to do what we've asked?"

William and his wife decided to see a counselor about this ongoing problem in their relationship. The counselor offered some advice regarding solutions to help them move forward together, encouraging them to find non-verbal cues that would serve as the reminder and replace verbal nagging.

For example, William's wife would walk next to him and place her hand softly on his upper back to remind him about his stooped posture. This gentle and loving touch would remind him that he was being asked to stand up straight. She did her best not to say anything when observing him from afar walking with a stooped posture. She would find opportunities to walk by him and provide the non-verbal reminder. A physical therapist had recommended that William check his posture every time he passed through a doorway at home. William's wife would remind him of this repetition by saying "doorway" instead of nagging him about the posture directly. This one word was the cue that reminded him if he forgot to adjust his posture at the doorway.

When William's wife had difficulty hearing him or noticed that he was speaking too softly, she would give him a thumbs up gesture so that he could visualize the need to speak up instead of being verbally told to do so. They also purchased a decibel-monitoring light that they installed in their family room. This light would turn red when

William's speech was too soft and would turn green when he was loud enough. William could watch the lights at the far end of the room as his cue to speak up.

William and his wife admitted that they were not perfect in executing this new plan; however, the major reduction in verbal nagging and the teamwork involved in using these non-verbal cues greatly improved their relationship. William's wife put a lot of effort into remembering this technique. She needed a great deal of patience with him as well. However, she felt that it was well worth the outcome: she became a cheerleader for his success rather than a parent nagging their child.

Chapter 3

EXERCISE IN PARKINSON'S DISEASE

Exercise is Good for PD

There is no doubt about the importance of exercise in managing Parkinson's disease. In the Pubmed database of the National Library of Medicine of the National Institute of Health, over 150 randomized controlled trials have been published on exercise and PD. Almost 8,000 people with PD have been studied in these trials collectively. These studies have demonstrated the benefits of exercise for people with PD, not just for motor symptoms or non-motor symptoms, but also for longevity.

When we interviewed our patients with PD, we spoke at length about exercise. Overall, across the entire group, the vast majority of patients agreed that exercise was an important aspect of treatment, and patients were willing to accept the need to exercise. Over half of the group already pursued regular exercise, although the type of exercise varied greatly. We found individuals who regularly walked the neighborhood at a casual pace or walked the mall with a friend. Walking sessions might last from twenty to forty-five minutes, depending upon the individual, and the intensity was typically low to medium at best. We found others who attended a boxing class for PD twice a week or participated in a group exercise class once or twice a week and believed that they were fulfilling the exercise requirement. At the other extreme were people with PD who worked out for hours every day with moderate to high intensity.

> *Studies demonstrate that exercise improves*
> *the motor symptoms, non-motor symptoms,*
> *and longevity of people with Parkinson's disease.*

The younger patients in our group were much more likely to engage in an exercise program regularly. They were also more motivated to pursue medium-to-high intensity workouts as well. The older patients were slightly less likely to pursue regular exercise. We interviewed patients over the age of seventy and found that more women than men admitted they had no interest in exercising and refused to start exercising despite knowing the benefits. They admitted to never exercising in their life and did not want to start now just because of this diagnosis. Their care partner or caregiver had given up on trying to talk them into exercising and simply avoided this topic with them.

As we spoke to the mostly older women who refused to consider an exercise program, it became apparent that they were not going to change their mind on this issue. If your loved one falls into this camp and you are finding it hard to convince them to change their way of exercising, then it may be a lost cause. Hopefully, you may communicate the benefits of exercise and perhaps be able to talk them into starting a low-intensity program as a good warm-up before increasing the intensity, duration, and/or frequency of exercise. If the individual remains stubbornly resistant to the idea, perhaps it is best to respect their wishes and support them. When their condition worsens, I find that some of these individuals will accept a referral for physical therapy and that this private therapy session is usually better tolerated by the patient.

For the rest of the people with PD who are open to exercise and perhaps already exercise, as care partners or caregivers, our job is to support them in getting the exercise they need. Make sure that your loved one with PD has medical clearance to pursue the exercise program recommended. If you are joining them for exercise, make sure your healthcare provider has cleared you for the intensity of exercise that you choose. If your loved one is already exercising, then you can ask them if you can be their accountability partner. You can perhaps keep a record of their exercise for them if they wish and help them work toward their exercise goals.

There are numerous reasons why exercise is good for someone with PD. We know from many published studies that exercise keeps our bone health optimal. This is especially important as people with PD age and face the increasing risk of falling and breaking bones. Exercise has been shown to reduce the risk of developing dementia later in the course of treatment. There are also many cardiovascular benefits to exercise. Lastly, exercise strengthens our muscles, which weaken from PD over time.

When we look at the potential benefits of exercise for the Parkinson's disease brain, studies have shown that exercise has a number of beneficial effects. There appears to be increased blood flow to the brain, providing important nutrients for brain health. The brain's immune system is strengthened, as is its metabolism. Many studies have examined various growth factors such as BDNF (brain-derived neurotropic factor), a protein that helps support brain cells throughout the progression of the disease.

More recent research has also supported the idea of neurogenesis, whereby new brain cells are created in certain key areas of the brain such as the hippocampus. The hippocampus is a brain region known for its essential functions of learning and memory. A study using MRI 3-dimensional measurements of the hippocampus found evidence of growth within this region of the brain after one year of exercise, compared to a controlled group that did not exercise and showed no change over the year.

Exercise also appears to make stronger connections between brain cells by increasing the chemical release between cells of key neurotransmitters, increasing the density of receptor endings to receive these neurotransmitters, and creating more connections within the brain. As this happens, the connections between the motor system, the balance system, and the relay stations of the brain are strengthened. All of these changes lead to better motor performance as well as better cognitive function. Subsequently, mood, motivation, and behaviors may also improve.

It is important to know that many people with PD will experience a temporary worsening of symptoms immediately after exercise. A person may see an increase in tremors, more slowness or stiffness in their joints, and muscle weakness. A person may also experience an increase in fatigue right after an exercise session. The reason for this is natural in that exercise will fatigue the muscles and body, promoting the need to rest. However, this does not negate the benefits that will result from the exercise session for the days and weeks ahead, since the body and brain benefit from the exercise-induced changes within these organs.

A person with PD taking dopamine medication may also experience a temporary worsening of PD symptoms immediately after exercising because the exercise itself may shorten the duration of the dopamine benefit for that one period of time. Many people with PD are aware of this problem and resolve it by taking their next dose earlier than usual to avoid a wearing-off episode with their symptoms.

As a care partner or caregiver, it is important to encourage your loved one with PD to not be discouraged by this phenomenon and to continue to focus on the future benefits of completing the exercise session. As they build up endurance, these effects may lessen over time. Additionally, it will be apparent to the person with PD that they are getting stronger, enjoy better motor and non-motor function, and generally feel better about themselves in ongoing exercise programs. Furthermore, there will be ongoing benefits from the exercise itself.

We examined multiple studies evaluating PD patients in aerobic exercise programs of diverse types, and these have shown that the exercise program creates better physical fitness as measured by metabolic factors in the body. Studies have also shown enhanced motor performance regarding PD symptoms over time, such as tremors, slowness, and walking. Exercise has also been shown to improve off times in patients when the medicine starts to fade. These studies have also shown that longevity is improved in PD patients when they exercise regularly.

It is important for care partners to know what we are recommending as a minimum requirement for exercise when we offer these benefits. We recommend aerobic exercise for a total of at least thirty minutes a day, at least five days a week. This can be accomplished in one sitting or divided into shorter sessions throughout the day, as long as the total is at least thirty minutes. For example, some of my patients find that a fifteen-minute session on the stationary bike in the morning is all they can handle. They stop after fifteen minutes but then later in the day may go to a boxing class or Pilates class and add another ten or fifteen minutes of aerobic activity there to receive their minimum requirement for the day. Some studies recommend at least ten to twenty hours of walking per week or five to nine hours of moderate-intensity exercise per week. The exact type of exercise that one chooses does not seem to matter and we have not come across any studies that conclude that one form of exercise is better than another.

It is best to speak with your healthcare provider and obtain their recommendation on the type of program and length of exercise that is safe and optimal for your loved one with PD. And of course, if you plan to join them in the exercise program, then you should do the same with your healthcare provider to make sure you are being safe in your personal exercise program.

One of our patients had always enjoyed playing basketball and he did not let PD stop his interest. He decided to form a three-on-three team with friends of his age. They enjoyed playing and competing together and even qualified for the Senior Olympics. Each time he played he achieved his goal of aerobic exercise but did so in a sport that he thoroughly enjoyed. He and I are convinced that his dedication to this exercise is a crucial factor in keeping him going as the disease progresses.

Chapter 4

NUTRITION IN PARKINSON'S DISEASE

AS WE READ ARTICLES OR ATTEND EDUCA-tional meetings/webinars regarding Parkinson's disease as care-givers, we come across the topic of nutrition. There is a great deal of interest in the "best" diet that a person with PD should follow and much information about the idea of intermittent fasting and PD. I remember watching a recent webinar on nutrition for PD and think-ing, "I'm not sure what the best diet is to follow based on what was discussed."

Furthermore, if your loved one with PD starts dopamine therapy for their symptoms, the issue of dietary protein and how it interacts with the effect of dopamine therapy intake leads to even more confusion.

Despite all this, patients with Parkinson's disease are left with a personal decision as to whether to change their diet. Some people decide to limit their protein intake. Some go on a Mediterranean diet or MIND (Mediterranean-DASH Intervention for Neurodegenerative Delay) diet. Some decide to follow a ketogenic diet. Many just simply stay the course with their usual diet. Caregivers will often wonder if they should change their loved one's diet based on the information that they receive, especially if they are in charge of preparing meals and doing the grocery shopping for the family.

We decided to ask our patients with PD if they would like to have their care partner or caregiver change their diet and meal strategy for them. In patients with early PD, 71% responded they did not want their loved one to change their diet for them. Gender, personality type, and age made no difference in this group: all responded with a no. Of the 29% that responded yes, I would be fine with my loved one changing the meal plan, 82% were men, interestingly enough.

We then asked them if they were planning to change their personal diet plan to fit what they thought was best for PD and if they would like their care partner or caregiver to also change their diet to match. Interestingly, 85% of the early PD patients said no. For the patients that preferred their care partner to also change their meal, not surprisingly the majority were Type A personalities. Gender did not play a role in the response.

For the advanced PD group, we asked the patients if they needed help preparing meals. In our group, 50% needed help preparing meals (for both physical and mental reasons), while 90% did not need help with feeding at mealtimes due to the symptoms of PD. We asked this group the same two questions: would you like your caregiver to change your diet based upon the available research for Parkinson's disease and would you like your caregiver to also change their diet to match your PD diet; 84% of these advanced PD patients did not want their caregivers to change their diet. Again, for the people who were interested in having their diet changed for them, 67% were men and Type A personalities. An even higher percentage of these patients, 92%, did not want their caregiver to have to change their diet to match theirs. Of the 8% that did want their caregiver to change their diet, all of them reported being Type A personalities.

First Steps to Improving Diet

It is critical for the person with PD and/or caregiver who is considering a major diet change to first discuss this change with their primary healthcare provider to make sure it is safe for them. Certain diets may be unsafe for an individual either because of a co-existing medical condition and/or medications they are on. For example, a person with diabetes mellitus may need to follow a certain diet and may have to eat at more regular intervals to maintain safe blood sugar levels and to protect against dropping into low blood sugar episodes called hypoglycemia.

Ask your healthcare provider if you would benefit from consulting with a nutritionist. Nutritionists specialize in optimizing your dietary goals and can help tailor a specific plan to meet your needs. They can also help monitor your overall caloric intake as well as different macronutrients intake.

Is There a Best Diet
for Parkinson's Disease?

It has been particularly challenging to study diets in relation to Parkinson's disease. For one, PD progresses so slowly that to study the long-term benefits of a specific diet would require an exceptionally long trial, and scientists would have great difficulty funding such as long study. If you tried to retrospectively evaluate one dietary choice of a group of people with PD compared to another group, you would find too many variables and confounders that would limit any valid conclusions. For example, people naturally have a tough time staying with one particular diet for extended periods of time: people tend to cheat on diets, or often binge eat at times of celebration or times of weakness. A person may say they are following a Mediterranean diet but then binge on sugar-filled snacks or desserts, thus negating any benefits from that diet. A Mediterranean diet may mean one thing to one person and something completely different to another person.

Furthermore, people tend not to be completely honest when self-reporting their dietary habits. So, to conduct a proper dietary study, the participants would have to be in a controlled environment and studied prospectively with complete control over everything that is eaten during the study. Typically, this would be done in a hospital or research facility where all orally ingested items were carefully controlled, counted, and evaluated.

Despite these challenges, we have received some interesting study results in recent years from colleagues in New Zealand. Dr. Matthew Philips, a neurologist and scientist in New Zealand, and his colleagues, conducted the first-ever randomized-controlled study on a dietary treatment of PD. The results were published in 2018 in the journal *Movement Disorders*. (Low fat versus ketogenic diet in Parkinson's disease: a pilot randomized controlled trial. *Movement Disorders*, 2018.) A randomized-controlled study is the best study to determine if an intervention is truly causing the desired outcome.

Dr. Philips and colleagues specifically evaluated the ketogenic diet. In this trial, they divided the participants with PD into two groups. One group received the ketogenic diet while the control group received a low-fat diet. They followed the groups for two months. They analyzed the groups at baseline, at the end of the first month, and then again at the end of the second month in order to determine if any of the symptoms of PD were improved by comparing the two diets. They evaluated both motor and non-motor symptoms.

The ketogenic diet used in this study consisted of high fat and low carbohydrates. Meanwhile, the low-fat group were allowed to eat more carbohydrates but at the same time had a low-fat diet. Both groups had the same protein intake. The participants stayed on their usual PD treatments throughout the study. Forty-seven participants were studied. The researchers measured blood glucose and ketones in both groups. The low-fat group received negligible ketone fuel for brain metabolism while the ketogenic diet group had a constant diet providing the brain with 15-20% ketones for brain fuel versus glucose. This was evaluated as a mild-to-moderate ketone diet.

The results at the end of the eight weeks showed a clear difference between groups. They found over a 40% improvement in non-motor symptoms in the ketogenic diet group. The longer they followed the diet, the clearer the separation between the groups as far as these benefits were concerned. The control group on the low-fat diet did improve as well, but by only 11%. The non-motor symptoms that improved included urinary dysfunction, pain, fatigue, sleepiness, and cognitive impairment. These are often non-motor symptoms that fail to respond to the dopamine treatments used to treat the motor symptoms of PD. When they looked at the motor symptoms, there was an improvement of about 25% in both groups. This included slowness, tremors, and stiffness for the motor symptoms.

The investigators pointed out that longer studies are needed, especially with more people. It would be interesting to see if intermittent fasting, which may create an even higher ketone effect, would also benefit people with PD. Both groups also benefited from these dietary changes in that highly processed foods with high sugar/carb ratios as well as a multitude of preservatives were not provided to the participants. We can only imagine what type of benefit we might see in the progression rate of someone with PD who avoided pesticide exposure and other chemicals in their diet by eating more organic whole foods and less processed foods.

Best Diet for Parkinson's Disease

We still do not have the ultimate diet recommendation for our people with PD currently. However, the current data suggest that the MIND diet, which is a combination of the Mediterranean diet and the DASH (Dietary Approaches to Stop Hypertension) with the approach of intermittent fasting of food (but not water or coffee) or time-restricted eating, may be the best recommendation for PD. People with PD must make sure that whatever diet they are following provides adequate amounts of protein to prevent more muscle loss and weakness as they age and PD progresses. The timing of protein's relationship to oral dopamine medication remains important as well and is discussed in more detail in the next chapter.

We would recommend that you consult your healthcare provider and nutritionist before embarking on any dietary changes. Most people with PD that we interviewed stated that if they were willing to change their diet, they would want the changes to be implemented slowly to give them time to adjust.

Care partners and caregivers may be able to help their loved one with PD by following the same diet plan if approved by their personal healthcare provider to support the long-term consistency and compliance of their loved one. It is exceedingly difficult to prepare two different diet plans in the home, and it is equally difficult for our loved one with PD to adhere to a different diet as they watch a family member eating something they wish they could eat.

Questions to ask your loved one with PD regarding diet:

1. Are you willing to change or modify your diet to improve your symptoms of PD?

2. May we ask your healthcare providers for the best dietary plan for you?

3. Will you let me help you implement this new diet?

4. How may I support you with this new diet?

5. How much of the diet planning would you like to be involved in? (For example, choosing ingredients, planning snacks and meals, shopping for the food, preparing the meals, etc.)

Take Home Points:

1. People with PD tend to prefer not to change their current diet.

2. The men in our study were much more likely to consider a new dietary plan than were the women.

3. Most people with PD do not expect their care partner or caregiver to change their diet even if they choose to change their personal diet.

4. Consult your healthcare providers to obtain their recommendations on the optimal diet for you.

5. Consider consulting a nutritionist for both you and your loved one with PD to learn more about the optimal diet for your health goals and to make sure that both of you are achieving adequate hydration, protein, and overall caloric intake for optimal nutrition.

Chapter 5

HELP ME WITH MY MEDICATIONS

AT THE TIME OF WRITING THIS BOOK, there are no therapies on the market in any country that have been proven to slow the progression of PD. Although many trials are underway internationally, we continue to await such a breakthrough treatment. In the meantime, the main treatment for PD is a medication that treats PD symptoms. This medication is a precursor to dopamine called Levodopa, which was first brought onto the US market in the late 1960s and sold under the brand name Sinemet. People with PD now typically take this same oral medication as a generic medication named carbidopa/levodopa.

Today, the gold standard treatment for PD is carbidopa/levodopa therapy. This medication may be prescribed in various formulations. It is available in an immediate-release formulation as well as a variety of controlled-release formulations or combination pills that incorporate a booster medication. Carbidopa/levodopa may also be prescribed for delivery by a pump worn on the outside of the body which connects to a delivery system either inside the digestive track or subcutaneously. Many other medications may be used in conjunction with carbidopa/levodopa to optimize the control of symptoms.

Be Ready to Assist with Medication

We believe that it is important for care partners and caregivers to understand how this medication works and how it is dosed so that they can better assist their loved one. As the disease progresses, caregivers will need to become more involved in dispensing the medication to make sure their loved one is taking the doses on time and correctly. Timing becomes increasingly more critical to manage the symptoms optimally. Your loved one will need your help. Be prepared to fill this role and arm yourself with a knowledge of these medications so that you will provide the best support. Talk to the healthcare provider prescribing the medications and find out how they want your loved one to take them.

> *We believe that it is important for care partners and caregivers to understand how this medication works and how it is dosed so that they can better assist their loved one.*

The dosing of symptomatic dopamine medication along with other medications for PD may be complex and a real challenge for people with PD. Even with the best cognitive clarity, a person with PD may still struggle to keep track of the timing of dosing and the numerous times they must take medication throughout the day and night. Additionally, a complication or adverse effect of dopamine may result in what is called Dopamine Hedonistic syndrome. This problem occurs in a person with PD becoming addicted to the dopamine effects. This causes them to want to dose the medication more often and to take more of it to receive a euphoric feeling or "high" from the medication. We have witnessed patients stockpiling the medication in various locations around the house, in the car, and in other hiding places so that they can ingest extra doses at will. Some patients have even received multiple prescriptions for the same medication from different medical providers so that they could take more medication than was prescribed.

Terry's Story

Terry was in his late forties and had young-onset PD. He responded very well to the levodopa medication for many years, which allowed him to continue working as one of the leaders in his company. As the disease progressed, however, he had to take larger doses of dopamine to keep his symptoms under control. He would take extra doses of the medication at work to optimize his performance and to hide his tremors from co-workers.

Eventually, Terry was taking dopamine medication every one to two hours while he was awake and then multiple times throughout the night. He became addicted to the dopamine medication and craved its euphoric effects. In addition, he enjoyed feeling his tremor abating and his muscles relaxing as the dopamine hit peak levels. As Terry ingested higher doses of medication than had been prescribed, he experienced additional side effects, such as dyskinesia, which fortunately did not become bothersome. The main problem was that his higher doses created an intoxication effect whereby his speech would slur and his balance was impaired, as if he were drunk. This side effect would wear off as his dopamine level faded. But now he was in an inconvenient situation because in order to experience the euphoria he craved, he also had to endure these adverse effects at the same time.

I remember one day when he came to the clinic for his regular check-up appointment. I could not understand a word he was saying. I thought for sure he had drunk too much alcohol as he stumbled around the clinic, but when we checked his alcohol level, we found he had had no alcohol. I kept him in the clinic for observation and asked his wife to come in to help me keep him safe there. A few hours later, his dopamine levels dropped and we could finally understand him when he spoke. When Terry's wife and I talked to him at length, he confessed to all the dopamine medication he was taking from different doctors and to the hidden locations where he was storing the pills.

We then alerted the pharmacies to allow only one prescriber of the dopamine medication. I also informed the other prescribing physicians of the problem and told them to restrict all dopamine pre-scriptions to those I provided. Terry's wife now took control of the pills and dispensed each individual dose to him as I prescribed; she also kept the remaining pills locked up and inaccessible to Terry.

Desire of People with PD to Have Medications Monitored

We asked our patients in the early stages of PD if they were open to their care partner reminding them to take medication and monitoring the dosing with them. 58% of the people with PD did not want their care partner to get involved with their medication. Most of these individuals, not surprisingly, were Type A personalities and typically younger patients. However, almost half of the rest of the patients with PD were open to receiving help even in the early stages where typically the dosing of medication is not extraordinarily complex.

Most of the formulations of dopamine require frequent dosing of the pills throughout the day and sometimes even at night. Unfortunately, the pills on the market today do not last for 24 hours per dose. This would be optimal and hopefully will be the reality at some point. Until then, however, patients with PD must take multiple doses per day—and this is not easy to remember. We are all prone to forgetting to take medication as we get busy during the day. We may forget a dose and then, by the time we realize it, we have started eating a meal, thus forcing us to wait even longer to take the next dose.

I find that many care partners are surprised to hear for the first time during an office visit from their loved one that doses were often forgotten. In fact, the reason many people with PD have mood fluctuations throughout the day is that they commonly forget a dose or take it at a less optimal time. This is when care partners realize that perhaps they should become more involved and help their loved one with this task.

We spoke with many people with PD who strongly object to their care partner helping them with their medication and who become frustrated when their care partner reminds them when it is time to take their medicine. A good compromise would be to have your loved one set a timer on their phone or find another alert system to remind them when to take the next dose. Talk to your loved one about how much they are willing to let you be involved and exactly how they would like you to help. Work with the healthcare provider to make sure your loved one is taking the dosing appropriately and not overdoing the doses or taking excessive amounts to self-treat symptoms without the healthcare provider's knowledge.

> *Work with the healthcare provider to make sure your loved one is taking the dosing appropriately and not overdoing the doses or taking excessive amounts to self-treat symptoms without the healthcare provider's knowledge.*

Most patients in the more advanced stages of PD were ready to receive assistance with their medication. Fortunately, most of them were happy to receive reminders to take their medication on time and most were open to their caregiver dispensing it to them. None of the patients in this research program had been currently diagnosed with an impulse control problem.

The very few advanced PD patients that wished to be independent with their medication and not receive help were identified, not surprisingly, as Type A personalities. They maintained an ardent desire to remain independent by controlling their medication dosing. Such a group is tough to negotiate with and many struggles may ensue over this issue. I recommend discussing any concerns with the healthcare provider so that they may be able to convince your loved one to allow you to assist and to be aware of what precise medication is being taken and at what time. This may be the first step in helping them monitor their medication instead of just taking away control altogether.

These findings are important for caregivers to know because we may get used to our loved one successfully controlling their own medication for many years. Many of us may have no idea what dose of dopamine our loved one is taking and no idea how many total pills they take over twenty-four hours. Often, the problems that people with PD experience throughout the day may stem from forgotten doses or delays in taking a dose at the right time. These instances of mini withdrawals of dopamine throughout the day and night may result in a worsening of motor and non-motor symptoms.

We learned that the incidence of impulse control problems with dopamine may affect as many as 25% of patients using the short-acting forms of the medication. This may be further compounded using other adjuvant dopaminergic medications, especially a medication named pramipexole (brand name Mirapex) which carries the greatest risk of inducing impulse control problems for people with PD. As a care partner or caregiver, you must remain vigilant for any obsessive/compulsive behaviors or new behaviors or interests that are not typical for your loved one. Some may express a sudden interest in gambling at the casino or online, while others may become obsessed with certain tasks being performed repeatedly or may indulge in shopping sprees. Hypersexual behaviors may also be common when this side effect develops. As a care partner, it is important you recognize these behaviors and report them immediately to the healthcare provider so that medication adjustments may be performed to resolve this issue, as these issues can escalate quickly and result in major financial losses or damaged relationships.

We believe care partners and caregivers should become involved as early as possible in understanding which medications and doses their loved one is taking to treat PD. It is helpful to monitor the correct dispensing of these medications and, when any concerns arise, the caregiver should immediately become actively involved in monitoring and controlling the medication bottles and dispensing the medication to avoid any complications and fluctuations of symptoms.

What You Need to Know About Levodopa Therapy

The generic medication named carbidopa/levodopa is the gold standard treatment for PD. This medication once had the brand name Sinemet, while in some countries outside the United States the brand name is Benserazide. Carbidopa/levodopa comes in many different forms, including immediate release tablet, controlled released tablet or capsule (brand name Rytary), rescue inhaler (brand name Inbrija), liquid gel infused into the digestive system via an external pump (brand name Duopa), as a liquid pumped into the subcutaneous tissue under the skin via an external pump system (brand name Produodopa), or in combination with a booster medication called entacapone (brand name Stalevo). All these formulations provide plenty of treatment options for your loved one. Many people with PD will be prescribed multiple formulations of this same medication depending upon their situation. Stay tuned, however, because there are more formulations (and names to learn) coming into the market in the future.

The healthcare provider will prescribe one or more of the above forms. You will learn that some of the formulations may be given with food, while some work best if taken on an empty stomach to improve delivery of dopamine to the brain. Do not assume that you know which way your loved one needs to take the medication: check with the healthcare provider regarding how your loved one should best take their medication. If they advise your loved one to take it on an empty stomach to avoid protein interaction, keep in mind that protein in some drinks and snacks (especially dairy) may impact their response to the medication. You may just be thinking about avoiding meals and forget a glass of milk or bowl of ice cream ingested at the wrong time and then notice a drop in the medication's performance. As a caregiver, you have a terrific opportunity to assist your loved one in watching out for these interactions and in timing the medication away from the protein if recommended by the healthcare provider.

Which Form of Carbidopa/Levodopa is Best?

This is a common question that we receive in the office from both our patients and their caregivers. Fortunately, we have many different options, as every person reacts a little differently to each formulation. There are a number of medical reasons why one formulation may be better than another for your loved one. However, the best formulation is the one your healthcare provider prescribes and that accomplishes the goal of treatment. My primary goal is to always keep our patients' symptoms optimally controlled and to keep those patients in the mainstream of life.

Chapter 6

DRIVING SAFETY

RIVING A MOTOR VEHICLE IS ONE OF THE most frequent safety issues related to PD. Almost all people with PD will reach a stage of the illness when they can no longer safely drive a vehicle. Over the years, we have seen people who willingly give up their driving independence and turn over transportation to their caregiver. However, we also encounter many people with PD who adamantly resist giving up their keys. The issue of driving safety for people with PD can create one of the most demanding situations for the family to deal with and even result in strained or fractured relationships.

Early in the progression of PD, most people notice truly negligible effect on their ability to drive a motor vehicle. Some of the patients who experience more pronounced tremors might report that these tremors are more apparent when they are clutching the steering wheel, but this rarely affects their ability to hold on to it or to turn it when necessary. Some of the patients may encounter a slower reaction time, but again, in the early stages, this rarely creates a problem with driving and could be considered "slow driving typical of an older individual."

Lastly, some patients may start developing visuospatial changes in the early years. This may result in more noticeable problems, such as difficulty parking. For example, the car may not have been driven all the way into the parking spot, or may be too close to one side of the parking stall. Some drivers may inadvertently bump into poles, cars, or other stationary objects that were "missed" as they attempted to steer the vehicle.

Almost all of our patients in the more advanced stages of PD will have significant neurological impairments (either physical, mental, or both) that impair the safety of operating a motor vehicle. Medications prescribed for the patient may also have side effects that impair driving safety. Both motor and non-motor symptoms may play a role in the safe operation of the vehicle. At some point, these neurological changes will lead most patients to give up their driving independence, or they will have their driving privilege revoked following a medical report to the motor vehicle department.

Not all patients willingly give up driving, and this issue can cause a great deal of stress for the care partner or caregiver and family, often leading to arguments and animosity, hurt feelings, and rifts among family members. Thus, this is an important safety issue to consider in the context of advancing Parkinson's disease, especially for the care-giver, and one that affects not only your loved one with PD but also other people traveling on the road.

In this research project, we wanted to explore the opinions of people with PD on driving at the different stages of their illness. We first asked the early PD group if they wanted their care partners to monitor their ability to drive safely. Naturally, care partners and families will monitor their loved one's driving skills and come to certain conclusions regarding their safety. For example, an adult child might decide not to let their parent with PD drive the grandkids out of fear for the children's safety, even if their parent has not undergone a formal driving evaluation. This kind of decision may have been based on the family member's observation and "gut feeling." It should be noted that this decision to not let the grandkids drive with the loved one with PD is often an early warning sign that the loved one's driving skills are diminishing and that more active monitoring for safety is now required.

Early-Stage PD Driving Opinions

Overall, 60% of our people with early-stage PD reported that they would not be bothered if their driving skills were monitored by a loved one. Moreover, 40% of this group responded that they did not want their family actively monitoring their driving. This is interesting because one would think that people would want to be safe drivers and avoid doing anything that could be deemed unsafe and that might ultimately result in themselves or others being injured or even killed.

However, 40% of our group wished to maintain independence and believed they could monitor their own safety. Men were twice as likely to report that they did not want their driving monitored and, as expected, Type A personalities were twice as likely to oppose being monitored; of this group, 82% that did not want monitoring were less than five years into the disease process.

So perhaps these individuals opposed to monitoring did not feel that monitoring was necessary, since they felt they were doing fine at this early stage. The older the early-stage patient was, the more likely they were to request the active monitoring of their driving, especially if they were older than age seventy. However, healthcare providers and care partners should be encouraging our early-stage PD patients to receive a formal driving evaluation at a local motor vehicle department to ensure they remain capable of safely operating a vehicle.

Advanced-Stage PD Driving Opinions

In the advanced-stage PD group, 57% of our patients were still driving at the time of completing the patient questionnaire; 75% were men, but personality type and age did not have influence in whether they were still driving. Of the group of advanced PD patients who were still driving, 56% reported having no objection to the active monitoring of their driving ability. Of those who still refused active monitoring, most were males and Type A personalities.

Harold's Story

Harold was a patient of mine with a twelve-year history of PD. His condition was advancing and his family felt that he could no longer drive safely. He had been involved in two accidents, but fortunately no one was hurt, and he had damaged several vehicles by backing into objects or hitting parked cars in a parking lot. Although his family continued to ask him to stop driving, Harold would not listen and continued to insist that he was fine to drive. Moreover, he always had an excuse for the accidents, which of course he felt were never his fault.

His family called me numerous times asking me to please convince him, at his next appointment, to stop driving; I told them that I would do my best. At the next appointment, after Harold had taken a neurological test, I sat down with him and his family and told Harold that I felt he could no longer drive a car safely. He became noticeably angry with me, but I insisted that he was no longer medically capable of driving a car. I told him that I wanted him to stop driving immediately and to let his family take over the driving.

Harold continued to argue with me and pleaded his case, but I remained firm in my recommendation. Seeing that I was not going to back down, he became even more irritated, finally asking, "Are you going to write me a prescription that says I can no longer drive?" In my head I thought, well, if that is what he needs to convince him, then sure I can write out a prescription for him. I answered Harold with a yes, took my prescription pad, and proceeded to write that he was no longer capable of safely driving a car and should cease driving any motorized vehicle immediately. I printed his name at the top, added the date, and then signed his prescription, handing it to Harold. He looked at it quietly for a few minutes and then tore it in half and threw it on the floor. Without saying a word, he stood up, marched right past me and walked out of the office, telling the receptionist that he would never return to this office.

And indeed, Harold never came back to see me after this unfortunate encounter. His family appreciated my efforts to try to convince him to give up driving. I did report him to the motor vehicle department and they effectively rescinded his driving privileges. In a follow-up with the family, they told me that Harold had stopped driving after that incident but always reminded them of it and would voice his disapproval of my decision. Thankfully, Harold was off the road and no longer a danger to himself or others.

Asking for Rides

We then asked the advanced PD patients who were no longer driving if they had any difficulty asking and receiving rides from caregivers or family members when they wished to go somewhere, 45% did admit that it was difficult to ask others for help. Both men and women found it equally difficult to ask for rides. Upon further questioning, we realized that the difficulty was not only in finding people available to provide a ride. The fact was that many did not want to be a burden and so were reluctant to ask even the caregiver who was living in the same home. They did not want to burden them with one more task, so they often refrained from asking. Additionally, many admitted that their caregiver was not very receptive to driving them places and so they avoided any conflict by simply not asking them.

We received feedback from people with PD who have no difficulty asking for rides and accepting transportation when they wish to leave their home. They reported that their caregiver arranged for them to have a driver take them to their various activities. For example, the caregiver would arrange for other family members or friends to pick up their loved one with PD and drive them back and forth to certain events or meetings, and the caregiver would also take them to certain places. They kept the lines of communication open when it came to wanting to be taken somewhere so that the person with PD did not feel trapped in the home or limited in participating in activities outside the home.

We learned some valuable information from our patients with PD that may benefit care partners and caregivers in relation to driving. We learned that in the early years of PD, perhaps because the disease did not significantly impact driving performance, most patients did not feel that their driving needed to be formally monitored. As the disease advanced, however, more patients were willing to accept the active monitoring of their driving ability by family. Men were more likely to continue driving during the advancing stages of PD. A rather high percentage (40%) of those with advanced PD still refused the active monitoring of their driving ability. Such individuals are often difficult for their families to manage because even when safety issues arise, they may remain very resistant to having their driving objectively evaluated and thus to giving up driving even when they are no longer able to do so safely.

One of the ways that healthcare providers try to help families in situations where driving safety is under debate is to recommend a formal driving evaluation by the local motor vehicle department. This should not be a one-time evaluation but, importantly, should be repeated at least on a yearly basis or even more frequently if problems arise. The driving evaluation is performed by an officer or trained motor vehicle driving evaluator capable of assessing driving safety. If the patient is deemed no longer able to drive safely by the motor vehicle department, their decision will enable the family to step aside and avoid being labeled the "bad guys" who took away their loved one's driving privileges. On the other hand, if the patient is deemed capable of driving safely, this may give them some legal protection to continue driving, although both patient and family, along with their healthcare providers, still need to monitor the patient's driving safety. For instance, some limits may be necessary, such as advising the patient not to drive at high speeds on the highway or not driving in the dark or during suboptimal weather conditions. In addition, driving distance may also be important, given the possibly of the patient falling asleep at the wheel as a result of poor sleep patterns or the adverse effects of medication.

When a loved one with PD stops driving and their independence is curtailed, we believe it is important to communicate with them regarding their needs. Delegating driving duties to family and friends may be the best way to help your loved one while at the same time facilitating your caregiving duties. Do not assume that your loved one does not want to leave home just because they do not ask for a ride. This new situation of being unable to drive may be a source of significant stress for them; moreover, they may also be trying to avoid being a burden to you.

Chapter 7

COMMUNICATION

OF ALL THE ADVICE THAT WE RECEIVED from the people with PD in our research project, the most important by far was communication. Our patients emphasized that regular and effective communication between the patient and the care partner or caregiver is crucial to maintaining a healthy relationship. Ironically, people with PD increasingly struggle with their ability to communicate throughout the disease process. Many of our patients felt that they either struggled to communicate their feelings and wishes in different circumstances or that their communication was not being understood and/or appreciated.

It is important to be specific about your needs when you communicate. Do not just use generalities but provide specific needs to be as clear as possible. It is also important that both the person with PD and the caregiver communicate their needs to each other. Do not let this be a one-sided exchange. Both parties need to communicate with each other so that there are no misunderstandings or suppressed feelings.

Meredith's Story

Meredith had advanced PD along with severe degenerative disk disease of the lower back. The pain from the latter limited her ability to stand or walk for very long, while her PD made it difficult for her to balance and coordinate her movements. Her husband is her caregiver and the couple live in their home, while two adult daughters live nearby with their families. Meredith's husband has taken over the household duties such as preparing meals and cleaning the house.

I asked Meredith what her greatest frustration was with her caregiver. Without skipping a beat, she said, "I cannot communicate my feelings and desires to my husband. I do not feel like he would listen, and he might even get upset with me for what I might say to him."

I asked her what she would want him to know. She explained that her daughters would love to come over a few days a week to clean the house properly and help with some meals. She felt her husband was not adequately cleaning the house. For example, she would wait for him to go to the restroom after a meal and then try to wipe the table down properly before he returned. She could not sneak around to clean otherwise without him knowing, so she felt trapped, living in a home that was not being taken care of to the standards she expected and had lived up to during their marriage. She was afraid to offend him since he was trying to help so much. When she had offered her daughter's help in the past, he had dismissed her request and did not want to burden their daughters with work that he felt that he could manage.

Many other people with PD in our group expressed similar concerns. They would say they wished their caregiver would help more with certain chores or allow other people to come into the house to help them out, but they were often afraid to ask because they did not want to create more burdens for their loved one in addition to the caregiving duties they already assisted with.

In these difficult situations, care partners and caregivers have an opportunity to make more of a regular effort and take the lead in sitting down with their loved one with PD and actively listening to them. Try to ask them what concerns they have. What could I do better? How can I do a better job of helping you and our family? It is important to approach this in a positive and genuinely caring way, or else your loved one with PD may not feel comfortable opening up and expressing their concerns. Many patients live with excessive anxiety and frustration simply because they are not able to communicate their needs.

As caregivers, we want our loved one to feel secure and connected to us. People with PD want to feel validated in their concerns and to know they can trust their caregivers. If a person with PD has difficulty expressing themselves because the caregiver does not give them the opportunity to express their honest feelings and opinions, or does not care to hear their feelings, then the person with PD will not feel safe in the relationship. This does not mean a caregiver has to agree with everything their loved one says; they simply need to acknowledge the feelings and opinions expressed so the patient feels heard and appreciated.

Many couples have set up communication sessions to facilitate a healthier exchange opportunity. This may be especially helpful if either party or both parties tend to interrupt each other or quickly dismiss what the other is saying. These couples will sit down in a comfortable place, facing each other, with good eye contact and positive body language. They will set a time limit of three to five minutes and then allow one person only to speak openly and honestly without interruption until the timer buzzes. The person is allowed to speak freely on whatever topic they wish. When their time is up, the other partner can speak. Before the silent partner begins speaking, however, it is important that he or she ask any questions or request any clarifications about what was said. This communicates that the speaking partner was heard and validated.

If a couple attempts to communicate but quickly find themselves arguing, this may be because they are using language that blames or criticizes the other. Here it is recommended that the person communicating should try to use "I" statements. For example, "I really need more help getting in and out of the bed each night." The use of "I" better communicates one's needs, as opposed to saying, "You never help me enough when I get in and out of bed." Furthermore, you could try saying, "I feel _____ when_____." For example, "I feel angry when you finish my sentences for me and don't let me finish what I was trying to say."

Caregivers should plan to organize daily or weekly "check-ins" with their loved one as a way of reconnecting with them. This check-in time should be scheduled just like booking a doctor's appointment, or could be done on a date night, for example. Some couples will take a walk in their neighborhood and communicate during this protected time when there are no distractions. I would recommend adding a gratitude exercise at the end when each person takes a few minutes to verbally express one to three things they are grateful for in the relationship. This simple act can do wonders in strengthening a positive bond between partners.

If you or your loved one is struggling to communicate without causing hurt feelings or conflict, psychologists teach a communication method known as the 'sandwich method', whereby you place a positive statement on either side of your demand or needful statement. For example, "Thank you so much for lifting me out of the chair and making sure I made it safely to the bathroom. Would you please clean up the mess I made in the bathroom? I really appreciate all of the immense help you give me each day." Creating a sandwich of positive statements around your request or concern is more likely to elicit a positive and healthy response from your caregiver.

Some couples would really benefit from seeing a counselor or psychologist. If communication is a struggle, the therapist may be able to facilitate healthy communication between patient and caregiver. They may offer strategies to help enhance communication and teamwork. They may also provide a safe space in which to discuss concerns and grievances, and can help you work on techniques to achieve better communication and a better relationship.

Chapter 8

MY ADVICE TO YOU

William's Advice:
"Don't over-care for your loved one!"

William is a husband with PD who sat down with us to share some advice. He was diagnosed with PD about twenty years ago and was in the more advanced stage of the disease. He had no cognitive impairment but only advanced physical symptoms of PD. His wife of forty-five years, Betsy, was a retired second-grade schoolteacher. Betsy had spent most of her adult life as a mother to their two children and as an elementary school teacher, mothering her classroom full of children.

As his disease advanced, William experienced a worsening of his walking and balance. He had some difficulty standing up from the chair despite feeling "on" with his last dose of dopamine. As he stood up, he would take a minute or two to make sure he was not going to feel dizzy before starting to walk. However, when standing, he felt that his center of gravity was off and just felt off balance. As he walked with his body stooped forward and his feet shuffling along, he knew that he had to be extra slow and careful when turning, as he had already fallen countless times when deciding to turn at a faster pace or to pick up something off the ground.

William had suffered several major falls in the last two years. One time his body fell to the ground in a crash that sounded just like a tree slamming to the forest floor. As he could not react fast enough to brace himself during the fall, his head slammed into the tile floor, resulting in a three-inch laceration on his scalp. He suffered a concussion but did not lose consciousness. Betsy watched this fall from across the room; the bloody floor looked like a crime scene. She took him to the ER and William received eleven staples to close his wound.

On another occasion, William turned too quickly and fell in the garage after getting out of his car. He fell on his side, this time on the concrete floor. Although he did not hit his head, his arm took the brunt of the impact. William remembers the pain shooting up and down his arm, but he also remembers the look on Betsy's face when she ran around the car and found him on the ground. He said he will never forget how frightened she looked.

William did not feel as if he could stand up at that moment. His main concern was not his injured body, but rather he did not want Betsy to try to lift him up: she was a frail woman weighing only around 100 pounds. Many people with PD share this same fear of hurting their care partner or caregiver when they attempt to help them up from a fall. William insisted that Betsy call their neighbor to come over and pick him up off the floor, which she finally agreed to do that day. William accompanied Betsy to the local orthopedic emergency center to have his arm fracture diagnosed and to receive treatment.

With this new balance challenge for the couple, Betsy became much more fearful of William falling than William himself. She would follow him around the house wherever he went. She would even try to prevent him from getting up too much to walk. Unless it was absolutely necessary to walk somewhere, Betsy would try to keep him in the chair and run to get whatever he needed so that he would not have to get up. She was so worried about him falling again that the sound of his body crashing to the floor continued echo in her mind.

Betsy had turned into a helicopter caregiver. She watched William's every move and circled around him day and night, trying to be there to prevent further falls. Although William was slightly annoyed with her constant hovering, he had a different complaint: he was now being treated like one of her second-grade students. His wife had turned into a mother and teacher to William, instructing him on what to do and what not to do. She constantly spoke to him in a tone that made him feel like a child, and she became strict in her responses to him and did not tolerate any back-talk from him.

William shared with us that his greatest advice to caregivers is to avoid treating your loved one like a child and hovering like a helicopter parent. William understood that he had a balance problem. He realized that he needed help and was always willing to use his walker to try to prevent falls. However, he also wanted Betsy to trust him that he would try to prevent a fall just as much as she could try standing right next to him.

So many patients are worried about their loved one getting hurt in trying to catch them from falling or lifting them off the floor. William just wanted the freedom to try to do as much as he could independently and without being treated like a child. He was very specific about the tone used by Betsy, who would say things to him using a sharp parental tone and a slow cadence that made him feel like a child. This bothered him the most and put a strain on their relationship. His advice was to watch the tone you use when talking to your loved one and avoid speaking in a teacher-child or parent-child voice. He emphasized to us that people with PD want to feel helped, not helpless.

> *People with PD want to feel helped, not helpless.*

Jerry's Advice: "Give us a chance."

We interviewed Jerry in one of our advisory board meetings. Jerry had advanced PD. He shared the advice that caregivers should let their loved one do all they can on their own. For example, he said that when he tries to type on the computer, he often struggles. His finger dexterity is not what it once was, and he makes lots of typing mistakes as he goes along. His typing is also terribly slow. His wife would observe his struggles and try to type for him. Jerry became quite irritated with her attempts to help him and decided to tell her that he wanted the chance to do the job himself, even if it took longer and generated more mistakes. He also emphasized that he asked his wife to understand that he will ask for help if he needs it; otherwise, he will continue to try his best to accomplish the task without her help.

Caregivers often want to make life as easy as possible for their loved ones with PD. Jerry shared that it is easy for him to be lazy and ask his wife to fetch him a drink or do this or that for him—and she will. He said it is better for him to use his muscles and get up and serve himself. He wanted to continue doing as much as possible without being helped. He felt as if he would remain stronger the more active he was at home. At times PD robs people of motivation, so it is easy for a person with PD to ask others for more help than they really need. Jerry encourages caregivers to try to find a balance: help where it is needed but encourage your loved one with PD to be more active and self-sufficient during the more advanced stages in a loving way.

"Be patient with me."

Many people with PD we interviewed shared the advice with us that their caregiver should be patient with them. The hallmark of Parkinson's disease is a slowing down of movement. This involves not just a physical slowing of muscles, whereby it takes a patient longer to stand up from the chair and to walk forward, but also a mental slowing down. It takes longer for PD patients to think about what they want to say and to formulate their thoughts. There is often a delay from the time an idea is born in the mind until the desired words are spoken. One of my patients has an extreme variation of this problem whereby he pauses with a blank stare for close to 10 seconds before he is able to express the words he wants to say. In this case, it is exceedingly difficult to wait because with such a long pause, one is not sure if he is going to respond at all. His wife would often jump in and speak for him and then suddenly he would respond, catching everyone by surprise. He wanted everyone to be patient and just wait for his response.

People with PD continue to emphasize the advice to caregivers to be patient with them by giving them more time to do things and more time to respond. Helpful caregivers would wait for their loved one to complete their thoughts and voice them. They did not try to answer for them or anticipate what was going to be said. Loved ones just need the chance, and a bit more time, to get the job done themselves.

One patient emphatically reported, "I don't want people trying to finish my sentences for me!" This patient finally had to ask his family to wait in our clinic's waiting room. He wanted a chance to express how he was feeling at his appointments and to answer my questions about his condition. Whenever his family joined him for these appointments, they would talk for him and over him to such an extent that he could not get a word out during the visit. If I asked him questions directly, his pauses would make his family jump in and try to hurry the interview along. We found that giving him some alone time during the appointment to express his feelings greatly helped him, after which we interviewed the family to give them a chance to add their views.

Another patient said he felt that his caregiver was too demanding about him being on time or not getting ready fast enough. He advised just changing your expectations and being more flexible about letting him get ready as much on his own as possible. He wanted to start the process earlier so that he would have more time to manage getting ready on his own.

Tina's Advice: "Give me opportunities to experience joy."

Tina had advanced PD and was living with her husband at home. The couple had been married for 48 happy years. Tina had reached the stage where she needed a walker to move around the house. Her movements were slow and off balance. She needed help carrying objects. She could no longer prepare meals. She needed help cutting up her food and help with her personal care such as dressing and bathing. Her husband provided all of this help.

Tina enjoyed going to church every Sunday. Her faith was important to her and she valued the time she spent at church services. She also enjoyed the people that she saw at the church each Sunday and wanted to volunteer for the programs the church was offering. These volunteer positions gave her boundless joy because they enabled her to serve others.

Eventually, Tina's husband stopped taking her to church on Sundays, and for many years they seldom left the house. Tina's husband found it challenging to get her into the car and then in and out of the church. He would have to expend a lot of effort to help her around the building and make sure she was safe from falling. As his faith life was not as important to him as Tina's was to her, he was fine staying home each Sunday.

Tina told us that she felt bad every time she asked her husband to take her to church. She did not want to be more of a burden on him or want him to get upset or frustrated by the effort required to get her there. However, Tina wanted other caregivers to know that her situation, being stuck at home, robbed her of the joy of going to church. She wanted her husband to understand how important this was to her and to make an effort to get her to church on Sunday. She wanted him to let her volunteer for positions where she could help people in a safe way. For example, she could sit and greet people and do manageable tasks at the church on other nights of the week. She wanted her husband to find other people that could help them so that she could still enjoy these opportunities. But as she felt that her husband was just not open to the idea, she simply resigned herself to missing these opportunities.

Richard's Advice:
"Don't let me hold you back."

Richard shared some especially important advice with us. He and most other people with Parkinson's disease who have a caregiver do not want to be more of a burden on their loved one than they are already. Richard could no longer travel safely with his condition, but his wife still wanted to travel. She occasionally wanted to spend some time with family and friends outside of the home, but she was afraid to leave him or to do things without including him, so she stopped participating in these social activities. She also stopped going to the exercise group that she enjoyed, gave up her monthly book club meetings, and instead focused on staying with Richard twenty-four hours a day.

Richard knew that he needed help and supervision but did not want to be such a burden on his wife. "I don't want her to feel trapped," he said. He wanted his wife to be happy and to continue having the experiences she enjoyed. He did not want her to feel guilty about leaving him to enjoy activities with family and friends or just go out on her own. Thanks to respite care, they were able to work out a solution so that someone would stay with Richard while she continued to enjoy her time outside the home. He wanted her to know that she should not feel guilt or shame for leaving him in order to do these things, as it helped him feel better when she was able to enjoy her own activities. In fact, he felt guilty when he knew that she did not go out and enjoy those activities.

Richard said that for many years he took exercise classes with his wife. This was such an enjoyable time for both of them and he knew how much it helped them both. When he reached the stage of being unable to participate in their workouts, he wanted her to continue them on her own for her health. He said, "I used to go to the gym and I'd say, I'm going to the gym to kick Mr. Parkinson's butt today!"

Susan's Advice: "Get prepared."

Susan told us about a situation that developed for her and her husband. About a year ago, both she and her husband came down with COVID-19. Fortunately, Susan's symptoms were mild and did not seem to worsen her PD symptoms. However, her husband's COVID-19 symptoms were far more severe and he ended up in the hospital for several weeks, requiring respiratory support.

Susan was at a stage in PD where she could still be at home living independently without supervision. When her husband was in the hospital, her anxiety levels increased very quickly. She was not allowed to visit him in the hospital at that time due to a hospital policy requiring COVID-19 patients to remain isolated. She was so fearful that he would not make it through his illness that she waited by the phone every day for an update from his doctors and nurses. On one occasion, the hospital staff thought that he would not make it through the night. Fortunately, he recovered and was able to return home after a rehab course.

Susan told me that this episode made her realize that she did not know anything about their insurance policies, retirement, or savings accounts. She realized that she and her husband had yet to draw up a living will and to designate a power of attorney. She felt completely lost regarding family finances and retirement money since her husband oversaw all of these matters; she had never had an interest in any of them. This created further stress and anxiety for her during his illness.

When Susan's husband returned home, she talked to him about her concerns and they decided to meet with an attorney to gather all the legal documents they would need should something happen to either of them. Susan's husband then prepared some documents for her that explained all the assets and accounts they shared as well as how to access any financial information she might need in the future. He put together a reference binder for her and included copies of any documents she would need should anything happen to him. Susan felt strongly that families should consider organizing their personal affairs to avoid the additional stress involved in managing such situations.

CONCLUSION

CAREGIVING FOR A LOVED ONE WITH PD IS challenging, but it is a beautiful ministry. As family members, we are called to love each other unconditionally. Instead of viewing caregiving as a burden or a situation that robs us of our activities, travel, and dreams, we should realize that a caregiving opportunity may be far more fulfilling if we surrender to it.

There is no higher calling on this planet than to spend time loving a family member with PD. There is no higher calling than to sacrifice your time, sacrifice your selfish desires, sacrifice your travels, and sacrifice your interests in order to serve the needs of a loved one who needs you now more than ever.

So, where do we begin as care partners or caregivers for our loved one with PD? You began this journey by researching how you could better help your loved one with this disease. We did the same. The most important lesson that our people with PD taught us is the importance of communication. As a care partner in the early stages, work on building better communication with your loved one. Never assume that you know how your loved one is feeling. They may be hiding their deep fears and anxieties from you because they do not want to be a burden to you. Help them release those fears and anxieties: let them express them to help them heal and feel better.

Communicate with them about how you can best help and support them. As you learned in this book, there is a wide variety of answers to all of our questions. Not all people with PD have exactly the same symptoms, the same challenges, and, more importantly, the same opinions. You cannot assume anything. Get to know what your loved one is feeling and what they need. Let them tell you, "This is what I need."

In the later stages, you will be providing more hands-on care for your loved one. You will assume more duties at home and will take on more of a leadership role within the family. Remember that a person with PD fears losing their independence. They want to keep doing their daily activities and chores at home, and keep pursuing the same hobbies and interests they enjoyed prior to their diagnosis. Do not rob them of these opportunities! Do not take opportunities away from them in order to accomplish things—even if you do not think it's a big deal or an important task. Sometimes, staying quiet and letting your loved one struggle to complete their sentences and stories can be a great victory for them, even though you think you are helping by cutting them off and finishing the sentence or story for them. Let them accomplish getting out of a chair on their own, even if it takes four or five attempts. Resist yanking them out of the chair to speed up the process.

As caregivers, we also need to watch how we communicate with our loved one. It may be OK to 'nag', but we must watch how we say things, use the proper tone, and be helpful and respectful at all times. Do not bark orders at your loved one as if you were a drill sergeant, and do not talk to them in a tone that you would use on a toddler.

You will receive lots of advice from family members, friends, healthcare providers, support groups, books, and the internet. Often, however, the advice will be conflicting or contradictory. And this is to be expected because people have different personalities, different experiences, different abilities to manage adversity, different mental states, different tolerance to the PD medications, various levels of depression and anxiety, and different relationships with each other. PD is a disease that will also cause significant fluctuations in symptoms, sleep, response to medications, and nervous system function, and this will create additional variables from moment to moment.

Do not assume that the approach or method that works in your *own caregiving* will necessarily work every day (or every moment of the day) or for the entire journey. You must be patient and flexible. You must be willing to change methods as needed and adapt to the current situation. Communication with your loved one will help you navigate the unchartered territory that lies ahead. Continue to communicate and be open to change.

My Own Caregiving Transition

As a snotty-nosed, selfish teenage boy, I remember developing an attitude and teenage behavior toward my parents that I am not proud of today. I stopped showing my love to my parents, thinking subconsciously that I was too cool at the time to display that kind of emotion. In those days, I was a poor communicator and simply shared my limited critical information. I stopped telling them that I loved them.

Over the years, however, and despite my poor behavior and attitude toward my parents, they never stopped showing their love for me. They never faltered in telling me how much they loved me, even though I did not reciprocate their affection. Their love for me was unconditional.

Thankfully, my daughter, Felicity, did not acquire my teenage attitude and behaviors. She is the most caring young woman you could hope to find. She cares deeply for her family and for others. She especially loves to care for her grandmother with PD: she loves to bake her goodies and to spend time with her, and shares a meal, dessert, and card games with her every week. No matter how busy she is with her schoolwork and activities, Felicity always is available to love and care for her family.

Shortly after the pandemic hit, both my wife and I came down with COVID-19. My wife became extremely ill and was admitted to the hospital for several weeks. During that time, I experienced COVID-19 pneumonia. I remember having difficulty breathing and it was a struggle to walk just a few feet in the house. I did not want to go to the hospital because an adult needed to be home with our seven children. My older children stepped up to the plate and helped take care of the family and house chores. Felicity, in particular, kept me alive, making sure I could breathe, making sure I had enough hydration, and encouraged me to eat what little I could to maintain my strength. She instinctively showed love with a servant's heart for her family and helped us through this tough time.

My Dad's Story

My dad was the first in our family to come down with COVID-19. He was not only sick with severe pneumonia but also with blood clots in the lungs and required hospitalization for seven weeks. During that time, family members were not allowed to visit COVID-positive patients, and it was exceedingly difficult to obtain information from the healthcare staff at the hospital, even for a local physician. However, I was able to obtain enough information from the night nurses over the phone to keep track of my dad's condition. We tried calling him on his cell phone, but it was difficult to understand him through the oxygen face mask covering his mouth. Eventually, as he could not get help to charge his cell phone in his room, our difficulties communicating increased.

Several times during his seven-week hospitalization, I was called in the evening by hospital staff who informed me that they did not think he would survive another night. They asked me to get on the phone with him and say goodbye to him. Trying to say goodbye to my father over the phone rather than at his bedside was painful in the extreme, even cruel, especially during what seemed like his final hours. Suddenly, I was forced to try to express my feelings to him, share with him how grateful I was for all he had done for me throughout my life and how much I appreciated his unconditional love. I managed to get the courage to tell him how much I loved him each time I said goodbye for what I thought was the last time. Although they continued to predict he would soon die, he held on and did not pass away.

Finally, one day the isolation requirements were lifted and I was allowed to enter his hospital room. I remember seeing him lying in bed: he looked so sick. His body was so tired from fighting the respiratory illness and he had lost so much weight from not being able to eat. He had no strength to sit up in bed and had not walked since being admitted to the hospital. His bed sheets and bedclothes had not been changed in many days. He could not recall the last time he received a bath.

I was deeply vexed to witness my father's appalling condition. I left the room and found a nurse and several nurse's aides and sternly requested that they follow me back to his room. Together the staff and I gave him a sponge bath, changed his hospital gown, cut his hair, and shaved his beard. We changed his sheets and made him look human again. On his bedside table sat a breathing tool called a spirometer. He had yet to use it because no one had taught him how! I did so and encouraged him to perform some breathing repetitions using the device. Before I left that night, I gave him a long hug and told him how much I was praying for his recovery, and how much I loved him. We both cried together as we reflected on the traumatic journey we had both experienced.

The following day, my dad began a sharp recovery. He had a renewed hope that he would fully recover. He felt like a person again and was determined to work on his breathing and regain his strength with the help of the physical therapy team. A week later, I visited him in rehab and remarked on how great it was to see him sitting in a wheelchair eating at the table, with minimal oxygen flowing through his nasal cannula. Several weeks later, my dad resumed walking and was able to return home. That he survived is a miracle.

Since his illness, my dad and I talk every day and more openly share our feelings. Our communication has improved by leaps and bounds. We tell each other we love one another as much as we can. He tells people that I saved his life, but all I did was offer him the love and hope he deserved. Sometimes when we go through challenging times, we realize that there are blessings waiting for us in our moments of adversity.

Thanks to this journey with PD, I have grown much closer to my mom as well. Our relationship has changed. She also sees the loving side of me again. I check on them every day. I tell them I love them at every opportunity, and I say "I love you" without hesitation. Even though PD was a terrible diagnosis to receive for my mom and our family, despite all the negatives, the illness has also brought us some positives. This journey has given us the opportunity to grow closer as a family and for me to express my love to them in ways that may not have happened otherwise. PD enabled us to grow closer and to love each other more.

Throughout this journey, I have learned that there is no right way to be a caregiver for a loved one with PD. I learned you must use your judgment to process all the advice you will receive and gather all *the resources around you, filter the information, and apply it as you see* fit for yourself and your loved one. I think of the Frank Sinatra song, "I did it my way...." If you put the needs of your loved one with PD above yours, if you pour your love into your family member with PD, then you will be a successful caregiver. No one on the planet will be able to care for your loved one like you can. Only you can love your loved one with the deepest unconditional love.

All the people with PD that we interviewed for this book made it truly clear to us that they wanted people reading this book to understand how much they appreciate their caregiver more than they will ever know. They could never express their feelings well enough to explain how much they love and appreciate all the love and support that they receive.

The greatest gift a caregiver can give their loved one with PD is hope. Hope provides the strength to cope with the adversities they will undoubtedly experience. Hope will give them the determination to live.

A caregiver once shared with me his motto: "Always travel in hope." I love this motto and I have shared it with all of my patients and caregivers.

I now share all of this with you and wish you all happiness and love in your journey with your family.

ABOUT
THE AUTHORS

FELICITY KLOS IS A HOME-schooled high school student living in Tulsa, Oklahoma with her family.

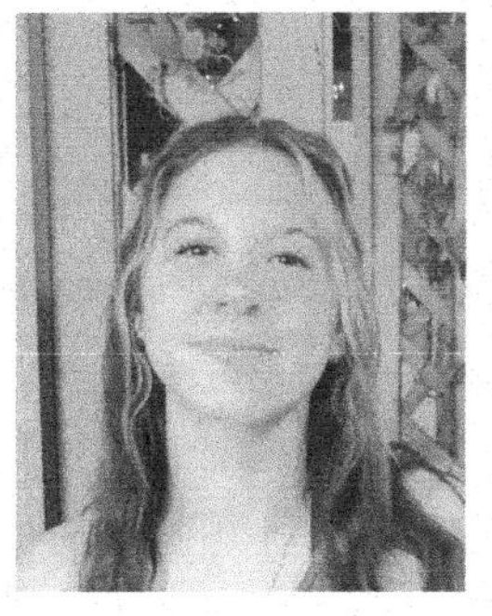

She became interested in being a care partner for a loved one with Parkinson's disease when her grandmother, Judy, was diagnosed with Parkinson's disease. Felicity loves spending time with her grandparents and baking delicious treats for them to enjoy. She made this book possible by helping to design the questionnaires for people with PD, facilitating the advisor meetings, collecting and analyzing the data, and proofing the manuscript.

Felicity enjoys a number of extracurricular interests including playing varsity basketball, painting, playing the piano, and spending time with family and friends.

D R. KEVIN KLOS IS THE founder and Movement Disorder Specialist of the Movement Disorder Clinic of Oklahoma. He completed his training in Neurology residency and Movement Disorders fellowship at the Mayo Clinic in Rochester, Minnesota. He has a large clinical practice in Tulsa caring for over 2000 people with Parkinson's disease traveling from a five-state region. Dr. Klos's practice includes medical management of symptoms, management of infusion pumps and deep brain stimulation therapy.

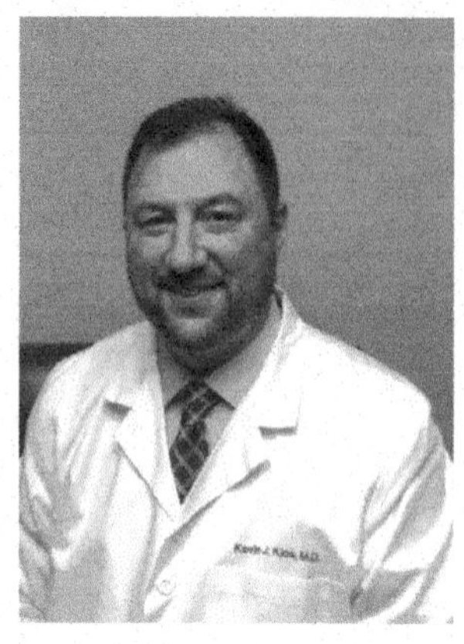

He is a principal investigator for international research studies in Parkinson's disease designed to find new therapeutics for disease modification and symptomatic relief.

He is the author of "You are a Better Parkinson's Disease Caregiver than You Think." (2020) Dr. Klos is a speaker nationally on research advances in Parkinson's disease as well as caregiving for loved ones with Parkinson's disease. He has first-hand experience with caregiving for a loved one with Parkinson's disease with his mom, Judy, who has battled the disease for over 10 years. He hosts a podcast for caregivers of loved ones with Parkinson's disease.

His mission is to bring better treatment solutions to people with Parkinson's disease and to equip care partners and caregivers to better care for their loved ones.

Visit **www.pdcaring.com** *for more information.*